I0467628

HELP!
MY PRACTICE SUCKS

HOW TO TURN YOUR FAILING PRACTICE INTO A PROFIT CENTER WITH FANS THAT GENEROUSLY PAY YOU

By Dr. Veronica Anderson MD

Copyright 2017 Dr. Veronica Anderson MD

All Rights Reserved. No part of this book may be reproduced in any form or by any means, electronic or mechanical, including photocopying, recording, or by any information storage and retrieval system, without permission in writing from the publisher.

Published by Dr. Veronica Anderson MD

Disclaimer: When addressing financial matters, we've taken every effort to ensure we accurately represent our programs and their ability to improve your life or grow your business. However, there is no guarantee that you will get any results or earn any money using any of our ideas, tools, strategies or recommendations, and we do not purport any "get rich schemes". Nothing in this book is a promise or guarantee of earnings. Your level of success in attaining similar results is dependent upon several factors including your skill, knowledge, ability, dedication, business savvy, network, and financial situation, to name a few. Because these factors differ per individuals, we cannot and do not guarantee your success, income level, or ability to earn revenue. You alone are responsible for your actions and results in life and business. Any forward-looking statements outlined in our book, or any other Medicine World Enterprises LLC materials, are simply our opinion and thus are not guarantees or promises for actual performance. It should be clear to you that, by law, we make no guarantees that you will achieve any results from our ideas or models presented, and we offer no professional legal, medical, psychological, or financial advice. If legal advice or other expert assistance is required, the services of a competent professional should be sought.

The education and information presented herein is intended for a general audience and does not purport to be, nor should it be construed as, specific advice tailored to any individual.

Intellectual Property Disclaimers: All trademarks, service marks, registered trademarks, registered service marks, product names, company names, published works, and publisher names cited herein are the property of their respective owners and do not infringe any patent, trademark, copyright, license, or any other proprietary right of any third party.

SPECIAL OFFER

Help! My Practice Sucks Bonus:

- Free One-On-One Consultation
  Spend 20-30 minutes working together to
  create a plan for your practice
- Everyone who applies for a consultation
  receives a gift

4 WAYS TO REGISTER

Mobile Text

Text to: 58885 your name and email with the
keyword **Practice**

Voice

Call 866-603-3995 PIN # 145733

Web www.Helpmypracticesucks.com

QR Code

Table of Contents

Introduction

Welcome to Help! My Practice Sucks. This book is dedicated to all my colleagues and fellow doctors who feel like they've got to the point in their life where their practice sucks. I've been there, done that. I practiced ophthalmology, started my own practice from patient zero, and got to the point where I loved my patients but I hated the practice of medicine. I hated the paperwork. I hated trying to get paid and feeling like I was not appreciated. I hated when people argued with my front desk over ten dollar co-pays, yet would go into my optical dispensary and spend seven hundred dollars on glasses -and then drive away in a Mercedes Benz®.

Help! My Practice Sucks is for all the doctors out there who have experienced the frustration of working those hundred hour weeks and feeling that they want something different.

So, let's talk about how this book is to be used. First, this is a combination of many years of practice and my entrepreneurial training, engaging with coaches who know about business. This book incorporates the fundamentals of business and approaches that any practice can implement.

Start with the mindset that, in order to have patients and clients who will pay you, they have to know, like, and trust you, and also value what you have to offer them. In addition, you must stand out from the crowd. Your services must be seen as so valuable, they are worth throwing away the insurance card and going with you.

This book is about how to differentiate yourself and provides some of the keys to setting up your practice. This is not a step-by-step how-to book with every single detail in it. This is a more of a concept book with points at the end of each chapter that you can implement immediately. Some of the principles taught in this book are going to be foreign to you, and some of the them may, at first, seem unnecessary or unrealistic to you. If you think that, because you're a doctor,you're above marketing and branding, then I encourage you to read this book with an open mind. You may not incorporate the things I suggest, but it may give you a foundation to think creatively about what seems right for your practice.

As you start out, embrace the interactive design of this book. It was written with your active participation in mind. There are links with what we refer to as "calls to action" in them. They are there purposely because I want you to take action and immediately start seeing results with each step, even when your practice is not the way you want. There are lots of opportunities in the book for you to start on this pathway right away. The universe loves action - so, when you get an idea, implement it now and then go on to the next chapter.

Second, this book is for the business of you and your practice. It's not clinical at all. You already know how to treat your patients well. You're a doctor and you're well-trained. You know what you're doing. What you will learn in this book is effective business strategies and what makes a good business.

Third, this book is for people who are implementers, and not for people who want to sit back and criticize. Only for people who are really ready to learn. Implementers.

Fourth, this book is not meant to be perfect grammatically or a New York Times™ best-seller. This book is meant to help you actually see and get results. You must begin with the building blocks. If you find grammar or spelling mistakes in the book, please send them in but don't get hung up on it. Those who do are using that as an excuse to procrastinate. So, if you're thinking, "Well, she's a doctor, she should write everything correctly", you're wasting time. Don't.

Next, realize that, although this book has a lot of ideas in it, you're going to need help. And I'm going to give you opportunities throughout the book where you can engage with me for that help. I wish there had been somebody there for me when I needed help with my practice. I wish there had been other doctors there to help me implement, doctors who understood business as well as the stress of being in charge of other people's lives. Way down the line, I found people who could help me, although most of them have not been people in the medical field.

Also, understand that we live in dynamic times, where marketing strategies are changing every day. Some of what I say in this book may have been true at the time the book was written but has changed with the evolving market. In the era of social media, what is popular at the moment may not be popular at the time that you actually read this book. So I encourage you to visit my website, where you will continue to find regular updates for this book along with new content you can use to engage and find ideas on getting people to know, like, and trust you – and to become actual paying clients.

I'm looking forward to getting to know you better. I definitely would like to hear your stories. I want you to use this book to learn how to think differently. What makes companies like Apple, Disney, and Ritz Carlton great? And what makes us all want use their products? Our mutual goal in this book is to teach you how to improve your "practice experience" so that you create a business you can enjoy and effectively optimize with clients who value every interaction with you. I'm Dr. Veronica Anderson and you can find me at HelpMyPracticeSucks.com.

My Story

In ten years as an Ophthalmologist and Glaucoma specialist, and owner of Eye Associates of Central New Jersey, I built a practice of over 11,000 patients using a simple motto that can be interpreted either medically or metaphorically: "Good vision improves your outlook."

Born in New Jersey, I received an undergraduate Bachelors degree from Princeton University. I remember the key moment when I realized how grateful I was to have changed my career focus from OBGYN to my later surgical sub specialty. That day, I was taking out a cataract from the eye of a gentleman who was totally blind in the other eye and couldn't see me at all. He said, 'Oh, my God, you're so beautiful, and you're a black woman, too! He had perfect vision in that eye and suddenly had a new lease on life. It was a fabulous day.

Triumphant moments like that aside, I realized shortly after launching my own practice at 31 that being an ophthalmologist wasn't how I wanted to spend my whole life. I knew from the age of four that I was destined to be a doctor, and I spent my whole adult life in a crazy whirlwind of college, med school and 100-hour work weeks — all the while juggling a marriage and raising young children. No one in med school had taught me anything about the financial realities of building a business from scratch.

As my personal and office expenses rose, my only recourse was to raise fees and find more patients— but even then, my income was limited based on insurance payments. The clinical challenges and emotional toll proved heavy as I dealt with severe diseases. While I loved helping people, I felt trapped. Clinical depression set in. Reaching a breaking point, I decided that the benefits simply didn't outweigh the risks. So I took the bold step of letting go of one life-long dream to embrace a new one, leaving behind my marriage, mainstream religion, and my career in clinical medicine.

Since that momentous decision, I have been described as a smart and outspoken, fun-loving voice for healthy living in a variety of media outlets. I apply my life experiences, knowledge of science, and educational and medical background to help improve the lives of thousands of people in a different way. I have integrated innate skills in clairvoyance and clair-cognizance into my work and provide Medical Intuitive Readings. And, I have brought into my new practice, skills in homeopathy to guide clients to healing and optimal health.

Chapter 1: I'M GOING TO MAKE YOU LOVE ME!

Would you be insulted if I told you to become a Mickey Mouse Doctor?

Well, don't be. Because it's a *good* thing.

That's because I define a "Mickey Mouse Doctor" as a medical professional who incorporates the outstanding customer service principles that make the Disney name magical. Those principles started with the man himself, Walt Disney, who put everything into not only delivering the highest possible level of product to his public, but also the best possible *experience* while enjoying it.

His first animated film, "*Snow White and the Seven Dwarves*," was scoffed at by the movie industry when it was in production. They called it "Disney's Folly," claiming that no one would pay to sit through a full-length cartoon about a fairy tale. As costs ballooned, Walt spent all that he had and then borrowed more to make sure it had a breakthrough level of quality - to the point where he mortgaged his own *house* to make sure it was completed as he wanted it to be.

That same care and dedication went into his theme parks, beginning with Disneyland, which opened in 1955. Again, he stretched his finances so far that he was forced to make a deal to produce the first Disney TV show for the fledging ABC TV network in order to obtain the necessary funding to complete the park.

Alarm bells ringing in your head? Are you saying to yourself, "Hey, do I need to go into debt?"

On the contrary - I would never suggest you go broke for your practice. Instead, let's look back at what happened to Walt Disney as a result of his commitment to *his* business. First, "Snow White" made *four times as much money* as any other movie released in 1938. Second, in case you didn't know it, Disney now *owns* the ABC network. That's the kind of pay-off I'm talking about (and you're certainly not going to have to take out another mortgage on your home to do the kinds of things I'm talking about in this book).

My point is that Walt Disney put an all-out effort into everything that carried his name. Not simply because he was a gifted visionary, but also because he knew it was *good business.* People trusted in him, believed in him, and kept buying from him. And even though he passed away over a half a century ago, people *still* trust in the Disney brand.

All this happened because Walt was secretly singing in his head, "I'm Gonna Make You Love Me," the whole time he was building his empire. You should be singing along, too, as you build your practice.

Disney in the 21st Century

Let's look at how the Disney difference is put to work today when it comes to their customer experience.

When you arrive at Disneyland® or Disney World®, your experience starts in the parking lot. Pictures of Disney characters are used to mark various parking lot areas, and trolleys come through to pick you up and take you to the front gate. If you're staying at one of the adjacent Disney hotels, you don't even have to carry your own luggage.

The employees, or "cast members" you encounter have been trained to be "Assertively Friendly." They have a standard reply to most requests - "You can have anything you want. It's Disney." They'll even answer a question like, "What time is the three o'clock parade?" patiently and politely.

Now despite this, writer Carmine Gallo wrote on the "Forbes" website that going to Disneyland and experiencing all this made him *angry*. Why?

The reason is all the great Disney positives made him realize just how bad other businesses are at customer satisfaction. Why can't everyone treat their customers like this? He gives a small, but telling, example: at Disneyland, the park is kept spic n' span 24/7 - so that it's always "show ready." In contrast, there's a restaurant near his office that's definitely not "show ready." There's a lot of trash in the parking lot and, even though the food is good and the employees are friendly, he doesn't go there to eat. Simply because the owner of the restaurant doesn't care how the place looks.

What does this tell you?

You might be an amazing doctor, but if you're not giving your patients a positive experience, if you're not at all concerned with showing them, start to finish, that you care about them, you might end up losing patients instead of building a stronger, more vibrant practice.

The M.D.'s Golden Rule

Okay, but you can only learn so much from a theme park, am I right? How do you put these kinds of customer service principles into action at your practice?

Start with what I consider to be the M.D.'s Golden Rule:

"Do Unto Your Patients as You Would Have Your Doctor Do Unto You."

Many doctors consider their end of the doctor-patient interaction completed after the patient leaves the examination room, or wherever treatment is given, because the doctor has finished his or her actual obligation.

But the Disney experience is not about obligation - it's about *experience*.

An eye doctor who's a friend of mine, Dr. Frank Bucci, knows how to make a patient feel taken care of after the fact. For example, if a patient has eye surgery, he wants to ensure that the person has a good meal afterwards to aid in their recovery. He gives them a voucher for a meal at a nearby restaurant where they can eat for free (he, of course, has negotiated a lower rate at the restaurant for giving them extra business).

He doesn't need to do that. He only needs to inform patients that they should eat shortly after the surgery. But this simple gesture adds a layer of loyalty to the equation as well as positive word of mouth. Everybody knows Dr. Bucci is going to feed you after eye surgery.

Truthfully, this goes far beyond having a meal for Frank. He's a warm and caring person who loves his patients. And when you love your patients, they love you back.

Here's another example of going above and beyond the call of doctor duty. A friend of mine went to see another renowned eye surgeon, Dr. Eric Donnenfeld. His was the last appointment of the day, and after the appointment was over, my friend stopped at the front desk and asked the receptionist if she would call a cab for him to take him to the train station. Well, the doctor was leaving at that time, overheard the conversation, and said, "Don't call a cab. I'll take you to the train station myself, it's right on my way."

Now, obviously, you can't do that for every single patient (and, by the way, if you do offer a ride, make sure you have the right liability coverage on your car insurance!). But when you just do something like that occasionally, it makes a huge impact. Think of the ongoing value you gain from a patient like that telling everyone their doctor gave them a ride to the train station. People don't expect that to *ever* happen!

But, again, consider the M.D. Golden Rule - wouldn't you love it if a doctor did that kind of favor for *you*?

I want to tell you about one other doctor who did something remarkable in terms of creating a memorable customer experience. He does high-end cataract surgery and is one of the key opinion leaders in technology and medication providers in his field. That means he is well-compensated, not only by his patients, but also by his work with pharmaceutical companies and device manufacturers.

Now, he took the millions of dollars he made from his practice and consulting and built a three-million-dollar eye clinic in Lima, Peru. It's the most fabulous facility you'd ever want to see. With its state-of-the-art technology and a wonderful, well-trained staff that excels when it comes to service, patients actually travel there for the *experience* he's created. Not only that, but he also goes out into the Peruvian countryside to help poor people with eye problems; he brings them back to the clinic and treats them for free. He's giving back with everything he's made by providing an amazing patient experience.

And that's taking the Golden Rule to the ultimate level.

The BIG Secret Reason You Want Patients to Love You

Now, you may say you don't want to have to bond with your patients. You don't want to feed them, give them rides, or even validate their parking. You make a good living without having to resort to that kind of crazy stuff.

Well, there's another huge reason why you want your patients on your side - *they're less likely to sue you.* Yes, a big reason you might stay out of court is because you're *nice* to your patients.

Most litigation cases are not due to actual malpractice, but instead, because patients didn't think they were being treated fairly as *people*. Procedures didn't turn out the way *they* thought they should have, even though the doctor didn't promise them any miracles. It's more of a psychological issue than a physical one because the doctor didn't take the time to build up any sort of rapport.

Numerous studies back this up. One that was featured in the book, *Blink: The Power of Thinking without Thinking* by Malcolm Gladwell, looked at conversations between physicians and patients. Some of the physicians had been sued in the past by patients and some had not. After reviewing the conversations, the study group could actually tell which doctors had gotten into legal hot water and which had not. Doctors who weren't hit with lawsuits had spent more time with their patients (only three minutes more on average, by the way), and used humor and active listening techniques in their conversations. The information exchanged by the doctor and patient wasn't substantially different - the *approach*, however, was.

Another 1994 study looked at plaintiff depositions in malpractice suits. When the plaintiffs were asked why they had sued, they predominantly listed relationship issues with the doctor, including being made to feel devalued, poor delivery of information and a failure to understand the patient and/or the patient's family's perspective.

So, yes, making your patients love you isn't just about being a nice guy or even about building your practice. In part, it might also be about saving your practice.

To be honest, some patients are difficult and may not like you no matter what you do. My advice on these kinds of people? Consider referring them to another colleague - they could end up costing you more money and headaches than they'll ever be worth.

Making Your Patients Love You: Action Steps

How do you "make" your patients love you?

Action Step #1: Optimize Your Physical Office Experience

How patient-friendly is your physical office? Give some thought to these important aspects:

- **Parking Area**

Just as Disneyland begins its customer care in its parking lot, so should you. Is there convenient parking close to your practice? Does your patient have to pay for this parking? Can you negotiate a rate with the parking lot and take care of the parking for your patients? Think about taking care of this small expense if possible. The last thing a patient wants to do, after paying for the office visit, is to pay another fee on top of that.

- **Office Entrance**

Is it a hassle to get to your office? If a patient, for example, is handicapped or elderly and not able to walk well, is there easy access to your entrance? Are you located on a street that's too busy and difficult to navigate? Is your practice in a huge office building and not easy to find? Think about all these elements and how you can make them more patient-friendly (even if it might require a change of location!).

- **Waiting Area**

Virtually all doctors end up making their patients wait a bit before their appointments - so make that inconvenience as comfortable as possible for yours. Throw out the ten-year-old issues of "Golf" magazine and put in more current and general interest magazines. Have a large TV that either plays health-related videos or general entertainment or news channels.

You also want to make sure chairs and couches are clean and comfortable, and if you have patients who are children, that there are toys and books in a corner specifically set aside for them (so other adult patients won't be disturbed). Having a water cooler available for thirsty patients is also a great and affordable bonus.

Action Step #2: Keep Your Staff All Smiles

As far as your patients are concerned, your staff represents *you* in their interactions. If a receptionist or a nurse is rude, abrupt or just plain dour, that makes patients feel as though they don't matter - and worse, that *you* don't think they matter.

That's why you want to put in place firm standards for how your staff should greet, treat and explain procedures to those coming in for appointments. Remember the Disney rule - a staff should be trained to be "Assertively Friendly." That means smiling when greeting a patient, answering even the most obvious questions in a clear and considerate manner, and making sure the patient is comfortable at every step of the way as the appointment progresses.

Action Step #3: And Then There's You

It's all too tempting for doctors to put ourselves on a higher plane than our patients. They're the ones coming to see us for our help - and, since we know better than them, we must *be* better than them, right?

Well, even if we did happen to be better than them, it doesn't do any good to act like it!

You should always make a sincere effort to treat every patient like a family member (a family member you *like*, that is!). That means being considerate, patient, and friendly during the few minutes you must actually interact with them.

Frankly, most patients expect doctors to act a little high and mighty - and they're pleasantly surprised when, instead, they seem very down-to-earth. That puts them at ease and makes them much more likely to continue coming back to see you. When you display a *genuine interest* in their life and their health, you create a lasting bond.

And that, in turn, makes your practice thrive!

Chapter 2: DO A KIM KARDASHIAN!

In the last chapter, I told you to be a Mickey Mouse doctor - and now I'm telling you to do a Kim Kardashian. And hopefully you haven't thrown this book across the room yet so I still have time to explain!

Kim Kardashian is famous for ... what? Kind of hard to say. Her dad, Robert Kardashian, was semi-famous for being one of O.J. Simpson's defense lawyers in the former football great's infamous murder trial back in 1995. But nobody really knew who Kim was until ...

until her sex tape leaked out to the internet back in 2007.

Later that same year, "Keeping Up with the Kardashians" hit the airwaves and this reality show suddenly made Kim a superstar. She earned an estimated six million dollars in 2010 because of her incredible status as a media sensation. As I write this, she's married to hip-hop bad boy, Kanye West. Her publicity train is unstoppable - people pay an insane amount of attention to what she does, where she shows up, what she wears, and what she says.

So, again, let me ask, what is she famous for?

Well, since she's on a reality show, I'm going to be really real: she's famous for being famous. She successfully generated a memorable brand - and that brand, in turn, continually generates ongoing fame and fortune for her and her kin.

When you "do a Kardashian," you do the exact same thing with your practice. When you build a successful brand, you build an incredible, intangible asset that continues to pay off for you in many ways and for many years.

Of course, you'll probably be more comfortable with the concept if we move away from Kim and her tribe, and instead talk about doctors who have successfully branded themselves. So, let's do that. Think about Dr. Oz or Dr. Phil - they once had normal everyday practices and managed to use them to create multi-million-dollar media businesses that revolve around their daily talk shows.

That's where a super-successful brand can take you - to the very heights of popularity, influence, and income. You may not need or want to grow your brand to that extent, but to achieve the status of a celebrity, you do need to put some work into it.

Climbing the Branding Ladder

If you're saying to yourself, "I'm not Coke or Pepsi - I don't want to be a brand, I'm a doctor," stop yourself right there. Because the fact is, you already are a brand, whether you know it or not.

Raymond Aaron, the branding guru, proves this concept easily and quickly. He simply asks, "Who do you think about when I say, "Always late?" When you hear that question, someone's face almost certainly pops into your brain because we all know someone that is never on time and causes us to wait for them. It may be a negative, but that's their brand (and it could be yours - if you're making your patients wait a long time for appointments!).

You want a positive brand, of course. So how do you achieve that? Well, Aaron also talks about a "branding ladder" that has five steps. Let's go through the steps of that ladder, from bottom to top, and see how it might relate to your practice (or, really any business, when you get right down to it).

- **Step One: Brand Absence**

Being at this bottom level doesn't mean you don't have a brand - it just means you're not promoting it at all. For example, if you're a dermatologist, you might be interchangeable with any other dermatologist as far as people are concerned. There's nothing special about you (that anyone is aware of, anyway) when you're at the Brand Absence level.

Frankly, the clear majority of businesses exist at this particular level - they don't understand what branding is all about and don't attempt to leverage their own brand. Many of these companies still can do okay despite that, but that's about all they do - okay.

- **Step Two: Brand Awareness**

Maybe you advertise your practice a little to get your name out there. If so, you're creating Brand Awareness. You may not be giving people a compelling reason to choose you over another doctor, but you are building to this level. This may generate some additional appointments, but it won't build your practice to the kind of level you probably would like it to reach (otherwise, you wouldn't be reading this book).

One exception to that rule is when you use Brand Awareness in a unique, compelling and/or far-reaching way. I was just talking about dermatologists, and one, Dr. Jonathan Zizmor, who made Brand Awareness into a giant plus for himself. If you live in New York City, you've probably heard of Dr. Zizmor because he puts his ads all over the New York Subway system and has done it for years.

Result? He's one of the hundred most recognizable New Yorkers, according to the website Gothamist.com - even though he's basically just another dermatologist. Granted, he started advertising like this 30 years ago, but, according to him, it didn't take anywhere close to that long for it to start making him money. He says there was a big difference in his business the week after he started the first subway campaign - which is why he kept doing it for three decades.

- **Step Three: Brand Preference**

Brand Preference simply means a patient would rather see you than another doctor with a similar practice or specialty. But note, there are two "rungs" above this step on the branding ladder; that's because, while Brand Preference is important, it's not the be-all or end-all.

At the Brand Preference level, a patient might call and make an appointment to see you, only to be told by your staff that you're out of town for the next two weeks. The patient has a choice - he or she can either wait until you come back, if it's not an urgent medical matter, or make an appointment with someone else who's covering appointments for you.

At this branding level, the patient will probably go to the other doctor and not think it was a big deal. Making the appointment with you is preferable, but it isn't a must.

- **Step Four: Brand Insistence**

Here's the level where good stuff really happens, because your brand makes choosing you a must. This is where your patients *will* wait until you come back to town. Or, to use a soft drink analogy, this is the level where you go to a restaurant and they offer you a Pepsi®, but you're such a confirmed "Coke®-head" that you say "NO." You'd rather have an iced tea or water than have Pepsi.

That's because, at this level, the power of branding becomes much stronger than rational thought. Let's go back to the Pepsi-Coke wars. Pepsi has run a blind taste testing ad campaign for decades - it's called "The Pepsi Challenge" and you're probably familiar with it. Consumers sample Coke and Pepsi, without knowing which is which, and pick the one they like best. Most favor Pepsi - even if they are fervent Coke fans.

Lest you think this is a fluke, the same pattern occurs with other brands. For example, Grey Goose® Vodka was subjected to a blind taste test against two much cheaper vodkas - and those who took the blind taste test were all enthusiastic Grey Goose fans.

Well, Grey Goose came in last in that taste test (and, by the way, these people were all sober when they took it). Which means, judging by the test results,

Grey Goose is making its money more because of its brand than its actual product.

When you reach the Brand Insistence level, your brand takes on a life of its own. Your name trumps everyone else's in your fans' minds, simply because they *think* you're the best. Now, it's almost impossible to reach (and maintain) this level without having a certain level of consistent quality in place - but once you have, you've created an amazing future for yourself.

So - what could be better than that? Well, I'll tell you.

- **Step Five: Brand Advocacy**

Brand Insistence is great. Your best customers won't settle for anything less than you. But Brand Advocacy is even better - because those same customers also won't let anyone else settle for anything less than you! In other words, your patients love the experience of seeing you so much that they tell all their friends and family that they have to go see you, too.

The best real-world example of Brand Advocacy at present is the brand that Apple built. I myself own a MacBook Pro - and I firmly believe, if you're working on a PC, there's something wrong with you! That's because the customer experience I've had working with Apple products, including iPods and iPads, has been so awesome, I feel as though I have to recommend them to others. Companies like Apple get back 120% of every advertising dollar they spend; that's because they have their users spreading their branding message to people in their circle for free.

Brand Advocacy is what you want to aspire to. Think again about someone like Dr. Oz. Everyone knows him and everyone repeats his advice (which is another form of Brand Advocacy). People say, "I saw this on Dr. Oz" or "Dr. Oz says that problem is caused by so-and-so." That's because he is a celebrity.

Like Kim Kardashian.

Yes, I'm equating a doctor with a Kardashian.

This may not be a pleasant concept to embrace, but celebrity is all-important in this day and age. If you Google "Autism," for example, you'll find links to articles that reveal more about what celebrities have to say about the subject than experts in the field. Of course, the celebrities aren't nearly as qualified to talk about autism - but, when they speak, they get the attention.

And, when it comes to subject matter in your field, isn't it far, far better if you get the attention? Especially since you actually know what you're talking about?

Finally, consider the case of Dr. Sanjay Gupta, who happened to become a spotlighted CNN host and medical reporter back in 2001. Yes, he has impressive credentials, but in 2009, it was probably his brand more than anything else that caused the Obama administration to ask him to be the new Surgeon General (a post he turned down, by the way).

Doctors and Branding: Keep Away from "The Kiss of Death"

Before we continue, we first must address a major problem that exists when it comes to doctors and branding. Most are firm believers in something that trips up their branding every single time.

What's that not-so-special something?

Doctors believing they have to BE BORING!!!!!

BORING is the kiss of death when it comes to branding. Nobody pays attention to boring - and branding is all about attracting attention.

Why do most doctors think they need to be the upright equivalent of a sleeping pill? Well, credibility is very important to a doctor - and conventional wisdom has it that doing anything "unusual" could torpedo that credibility. "Oh, no, I couldn't do that!" is the usual knee-jerk response to something slightly outrageous.

Okay, watch a promo for the Dr. Oz or Dr. Phil shows the next time one goes by. Or even watch the shows themselves. You see them doing anything boring? I don't think so! And yet, people take them very seriously. They hang on their every word, as a matter of fact.

Let's return to our branding pin-up girl, Kim Kardashian. As we noted, she first became famous - or, more accurately, infamous - for appearing in a sex video. Normally, that's the kind of move that everyone in Hollywood will warn you against. They'll tell you that it will doom a career before it starts.

Instead, it made her profile "pop" and paved the way for her stardom.

Now, sex tapes are definitely not a good branding strategy for an M.D. (unless, of course, you're a sex therapist) - but you can keep your stethoscope on and still cause a stir. As a matter of fact, you don't have to do anything all that crazy - but you do have to think a little "out-of-the-box" to successfully brand yourself.

Remember that the next time you think you must be BORING.

Climbing the Branding Ladder: Action Steps

One of the big factors that really can jumpstart your brand is something we talked about in Chapter One; making the experience of going to your practice as amazing as possible. A great experience is what prompts Brand Advocacy; when people can't believe how great something is, they feel as though they have to tell friends and family about it.

You can't rely totally on internal branding, however; you have to connect with your community at large to create a strong image, generate positive word-of-mouth, and attract new patients.

Here are three Action Steps to make that happen:

Action Step #1: Put a Face on Your Brand

People buy people. You've probably heard that axiom if you've done any studying in marketing. Most successful brands have a face out there for consumers to bond with. Whether it's a cartoon tiger (Tony the Tiger for Kellogg's Frosted Flakes®) or a hot female racer (Danica Patrick for GoDaddy.com), the right face makes the right connection to the audience.

Now, you'll notice the two examples I just gave have nothing to do with the product itself. They just represent the product in a fun and memorable way.

Your practice could do the same. While Dr. Oz, Dr. Drew and Dr. Phil are happily on TV 24/7 representing their own brands, you may not be as camera-ready as those personalities. You may not be comfortable doing videos or personal appearances. That's okay.

It doesn't have to be you.

I talked about Apple's "brand power" earlier in this chapter. Who was the dominant face of that company for most of its existence? The late, great Steve Jobs. His personality and vision defined Apple and represented it to the world.

However, if you delve deep into the company's history, you'll soon discover that the person who really pioneered the initial breakthrough technology that put Apple on the map was Jobs' business partner at the time, Steve Wozniak.

Steve may have brilliant in creating computers, but he wasn't the guy to put out there to the public. Jobs, in contrast, had the personal marketing skills to sell the brand himself - and both partners agreed he was the best person to put out there.

You've seen the commercials with the guy who says "I'm not a doctor, but I play one on television?" Kind of the same thing. There may be someone who can represent you in a variety of instances - maybe a funny, bubbly nurse, a patient who loves you or maybe your spouse. It doesn't matter if the person can represent you well.

Of course, it's much more powerful if you can do it yourself. There's nothing wrong with getting coaching in this area so you can improve your media and personal presentation skills.

You can bet many of the biggest TV doctors did just that.

Action Step #2: Practice the "Art of Influence"

In Chapter One, I talked about my friend, Dr. Frank Bucci, and how nice and wonderful he is to his patients. It's his brand. And I also talked about how he gave you a voucher for a local restaurant so you would have a good (and free!) meal after eye surgery.

That's using the Art of Influence. The patients who get the free meal talk Dr. Frank up - even the restaurant that he's giving all this extra business to talks him up! The cost of those vouchers is more than offset by the marketing firepower they deliver.

It's the kind of approach that creates Brand Advocacy. You want to do things like this, that cause your patients to talk about you, other businesses to talk about you, your staff to talk about you and, hopefully, the whole community to talk about you.

Besides these small acts of generosity, you should make it a point to invest in new technology and keep yourself on the latest trends in your medical specialty. When you introduce a new procedure or new piece of equipment, you can say you're the first in the area to offer it. You can also easily get these kinds of stories placed on the local TV news, radio interview shows, or in the newspaper.

And you can tell your stories online as well. The most effective way to do this is through YouTube videos that sell your personality (or whoever you've made the face of your practice) and also explain medical issues in a colorful manner. For example, I just saw Dr. Oz illustrating how men sometimes accidentally pee during sex with the most outrageous set of props you'd ever want to see. But it didn't matter that the props were outrageous - he was talking about something that was a medical reality and illustrating it in a fun and provocative way!

Action Step #3: Practice "Reach Out"

When I wanted to promote my eye doctor practice, I would go give talks at a local senior citizen center. I would explain how the eye works, and talk about common eye problems that the elderly experienced. After the talk, we mingled and drank lemonade, and I would leave my business cards there.

Now, that talk only took an hour or so to do - but its branding effects continued for years. As long as five years later, a new patient might show up who still remembered that I had come talk to her and her friends on that night so long ago.

Again, that act of giving creates Brand Advocacy. You're giving up your time and you're imparting useful and valuable knowledge; they get to know you personally and bond with you. And they tell people about that "nice doctor" who came to see them.

That's why it's important to be high profile in your community. Whether it's your church, a local organization such as the Kiwanis Club, or a local government function, the more you show up, the more people will recognize you and remember you. Even if it's coaching a Little League team - how cool is it that a doctor does that?

That kind of personal service causes people to like you. And it causes them to spread the word about you, especially if someone they know comes to them asking for a doctor recommendation.

You'll be the one who's top-of-mind - which is exactly what you want.

Chapter 3: MILLIONS OF TALKING POINTS - MILLIONS OF DOLLARS!

Okay, so we've already talked about being a Mickey Mouse doctor and doing a Kim Kardashian. Maybe you might think those two chapters were a little beneath your dignity as a medical professional. Maybe you think it's time we talked about something a little more dignified.

Okay. Let's talk about boobs.

This past Mother's Day, I wanted to start a conversation about breast health, but I wanted it to be a conversation that would actually engage a lot of people. When we talk about women's breasts in this country, it comes down to either one of two not very pleasant topics - cancer or pornography.

And yet, breasts are such a vital part of the female body, and so important to its health. Why can't we have the right dialogue about them?

I set out to change all that - by focusing on their positive attributes under the theme of "I Love Breasts." I launched a corresponding website, www.ILoveBreasts.org, and also hosted a tweet chat for #ilovebreasts on Twitter during Mother's Day weekend.

And I decided it was important to have a little fun with it - including gathering the best breast art available (bet you didn't even know that was a thing, did you?)! So, amidst sharing Instagrams of giant sculptures of boobs and other delights, we also tackled some important health issues that were important to women.

Well, that tweet chat was still going on two weeks later after Mother's Day was over - and Pinterest boards were being filled with breast art - which included some grandmothers with some very unusual accessories.

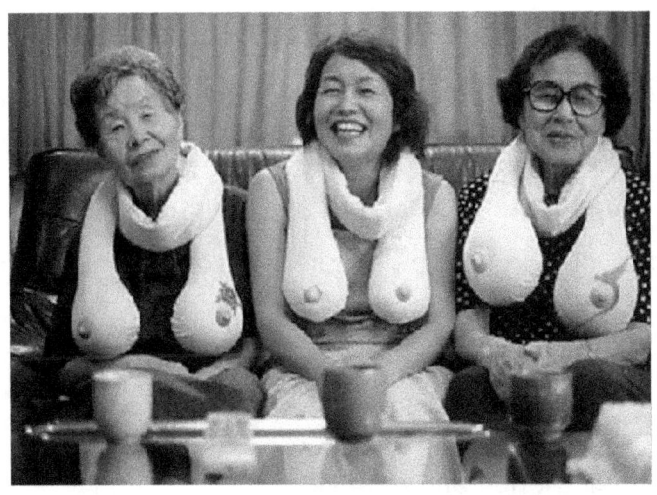

I got a lot of attention in a fun and crazy way. But you know what else? I was able to share a lot of important and cutting-edge information about breast health with my female audience.

And *my name was the link between all of these threads*; the fun stuff, the serious stuff, and the sharing of all these elements between my followers and their peeps. All of it fell under the "Dr. Veronica" brand - which made it a win-win for me as well as everyone out there who participated.

Even if *you're* a boob, you must see the value of that!

The Social Media Secret

Social media is an excellent way for your practice to get noticed - if it's used in the right way. As the title of this chapter suggests, there are millions of talking points you can use to ultimately make you millions of dollars - because those talking points increase your sphere of influence, transform you into an opinion leader, and engage not only your current patients, but also their friends and relatives.

But first, you have to do what can be an incredibly difficult thing.

You must get people's attention.

Remember when I said in the last chapter that the fatal flaw many doctors have is that they think they have to be BORING? Well, this is where that mistake can really kill you. Social media is like a party in many ways - and if you're the stiff in the corner trying to lecture everyone about diseases ...

Well, you're going to find your only audience is the wall.

Doctors can get away with a lot, because they are doctors. If I want to talk about breasts, I can do that - even though I'm an eye surgeon. But we all have a wide range of medical training that we can utilize in our social media dialogues. And you can use that training, as well as your experience and knowledge, to create talking points with power.

We've all seen people on Facebook and Twitter who post such mesmerizing thoughts as, "Oh, darn, it's raining and I forgot my umbrella!" or "Think I'll have a veggie lunch." Your practice can (and needs) to do better than that! We should be fun, but professional, a little outrageous, but still reality-based, to cut through the clutter.

Look again at the picture I included earlier in this chapter - the one of the grannies with the breast scarves. Now, that's the exact kind of social media image that people love. It's a little naughty - but, at the same time, the grannies make it adorable.

That's the balance you want to achieve.

Friending Your Way to Fame and Fortune

Many people attempt to put up a firewall between their professional and personal lives on social media sites such as Facebook. I think that's a mistake. For me, everything is professional and I don't bar anyone from being my friend. Why restrict it? I want as many people as possible linked to me, so as many people as possible know who I am.

Look, your friends already know and (presumably) like you - you've already got that group in place. What you're after now are the next levels - the friends of your friends, and even the friends of your friends of your friends (and the friends of your friends of your ... well, you know what I mean!).

Think of your social media presence as the biggest echo imaginable - if you say something that gets your friends' attention, they share it with their friends. If their friends think it's cool and something worth passing on, they share it with their friends. Your message keeps traveling without you having to do anything else. What you have going at that point is the viral effect that any pro marketer desperately desires - a free ad campaign with a huge impact that people willingly engage in.

Trust me, it works.

My Twitter group of followers is currently growing by 1500 people a week. Obviously, I don't personally know that amount of people - but enough of them know how much I have to offer that they say, "Hey, let me go follow her and see what's she going to post next time."

Going Beyond 140 Characters

Now, just status updates and tweets aren't going to get the social media job done to get new patients lining up for appointments. That means you should also be blogging, if you aren't already.

There's a good reason to blog about medical subject matter that you're an expert on, beyond your branding ambitions; frankly, we need more reliable authoritative voices out there talking about stuff. I noted earlier in this book that, when you search on a certain subject, you'll often unfortunately stumble into more celebrity rants than actual medical information - because

Hollywood stars simply get paid more attention to by the media.

When you blog, however, your content is forced to be recognized by that online god known as Google - and suddenly, you can start to become a big part of the conversation as well.

As a matter of fact, you can use that kind of celebrity misinformation to your advantage. If someone's popping off about something and they don't know what in hell they're talking about, you just write a short blog explaining how and why they're wrong. Because the celebrity's name is in your piece, it helps your blog gain more power with the search engines.

Of course, maybe you're intimidated by the notion of blogging. You don't have to be. First of all, you don't have to write long, academic treatises on medical conditions - actually, you don't WANT to, because most of your readers won't even understand what you're talking about! No, you want to take a much simpler approach. Here are a few pointers on how best to approach the blogging experience.

- **Do FAQs First**

Think about the questions your patients ask you repeatedly. How valuable would it be to them (and to you, for that matter), to start answering them with blogs you can refer them to on your website? You can also, of course, send out links to them on Twitter, LinkedIn and Facebook. If they are truly Frequently Asked Questions - a lot of other people will be interested in the answers, too!

- **Keep It Short and Simple**

A lot of people stop before they start blogging just because they imagine having to write long cumbersome pieces that will eat up all their extra time. It not only doesn't have to be like that, it *shouldn't* be like that. As much as you don't want to write something that's a thousand words, people don't want to have to read them either!

Two or three short paragraphs should usually get the job done, and the result will be a blog post that more people will read. If you are writing about something complex that requires more explanation, consider breaking up the blog post into two or three parts (as many experts do).

To really simplify the process, it's easiest to write opinion pieces that don't require a lot of research, but if you do need material that backs up what you're saying, you can always *link* to another online article for reference, so you don't have to go and on explaining yourself.

So, let The New Yorker print thirty pages about an obscure subject. You should be writing short punchy blogs about things people care about.

- **Lighten Up on Language**

You also shouldn't be using the *vocabulary* that *The New Yorker* uses - or that you likely use in everyday life. Remember that you're more educated that the average person; I'm not being a snob when I say that, it just happens to be the truth. Therefore, use language that's at around a sixth-grade level. You generally don't need a lot of ten dollar words to make your point - if you do, your readership won't even *understand* your point!

- **Go After Guest Bloggers**

One thing I do to increase my blog output is to invite guest bloggers to discuss subjects on my popular blog site. You can do the same. This doesn't make you look lazy or like you're trying to get out of writing something yourself; instead, it makes you look like you have a powerful circle of knowledgeable friends. That, in turn, helps your brand and lifts your prestige level.

Consistent blogging, by both you and your guests, makes you a focal point for information both in your field and in other health areas. By posting interesting and topical material, your friends and fans begin to look to you to keep them in the loop on what they should know - and, by the way, if you are posting an article or blog from another source, try to comment on it and put your own spin on it, so you can "own" it to a greater degree.

Succeeding in Social Media: Action Steps

Social media is the perfect place to build on existing relationships as well as expand your brand and build your credibility - without ever leaving your office or home. When you're a busy medical professional, you can't beat the social media combo of professional opportunities and personal connections.

Here are three action steps to make you a social media master!

Action Step #1: Be More Than a Doctor

Yes, yes, I know, you went to school for x amount of years and also went x amount into debt - just so you could be a doctor. Well, everyone can tell you are by that "Dr." in front of your name - and you shouldn't limit your social media presence to that aspect of yourself.

It's more than fine to show yourself as a human being, it's critical to successful social media engagement. The more people see you as flesh and blood, the more relatable you'll be and the more they'll feel "bonded" to you.

So, talk about your interests and hobbies. If your kid gets a big hit in a baseball game or graduates from middle school, post a picture and a comment. Talk about the sports teams you follow or the TV shows and movies you like. If someone disagrees with you, be good-natured about the debate. Show yourself to be a caring, empathetic individual as well as a knowledgeable professional, and people will respect and respond to you in a more powerful and lasting way.

Action Step #2: Make It a Habit

You must think about social media the way you'd think about hammering a nail into a piece of wood - you have to repeat the action, consistently, with the right amount of strength, before you're going to get that nail all the way in.

That means not just posting a status update about your dog every three months. That means taking *constant, daily action* that has an end game in mind.

Here's a typical social media plan of attack you might consider:

- Update Facebook status at least once a day
- Send out a tweet at least once a day
- Blog weekly. Link to blog on Facebook, Twitter and LinkedIn

- Solicit patient questions and comments on a topic once a month
- Post photos of weekend activities every Monday

Now, none of these activities, with the exception of the blogging, is only going to take you more than a couple of minutes a day - and the blog, if you think about it in advance, should only take you fifteen minutes or so to write, if you remember to keep it simple.

Those few minutes, however, will result in generating *a clear and consistent social media presence* - especially if you put even more time into making your posts as memorable and attention-getting as possible.

Keep in mind that there are social media coaches who can help you make the biggest online splash possible. They'll help train you to the point where your social media skills will be ingrained - and you'll automatically know how to use these sites to the max.

Action Step #3: Show Your Stuff

Let's say you're a dentist - and you see some friend of yours post on Facebook that they have a dental problem.

Make a comment. Offer advice. Nothing that would make you liable for anything, of course, but _share your expertise._

Social media is a great place to "show your stuff" in front of the whole world. Open up topics for discussion on Twitter, as I did with breast health. Create Facebook groups about areas you're expert in. Post little-known facts.

Put yourself at the center of the conversation about your primary practice area.

The more you demonstrate your expertise, the more credible you seem and the more knowledgeable you seem. People say, "Did you see what Dr. Smith said? Wow, he really knows what he's talking about," and your profile continues to rise.

Think of yourself in the same league as Dr. Oz and Dr. Phil. Approach social media as if you're that kind of media expert who people trust and turn to. Act the part and you *are* the part; after all, you are a medical expert, so it's not as if you're pretending to be someone you're not. Think of it as being like a singer learning how to perform in front of a crowd - it's a matter of being comfortable in that setting, not a question of having the talent in the first place.

When you create a million talking points, you get a million people talking about you. The more you make social media a priority, the more fame you garner. You want touch points constantly on Facebook - because, frankly, it's ultimately worth a billion dollars of free publicity - so log in and post away to achieve a super social media status!

Chapter 4: GIVE 'EM THE 411 - AND MAKE IT A 911

There's something I'd like you to do before you continue reading this chapter.

Go to Amazon.com. Type "Dr. Oz" into the online retailer's search engine box and see how many related product results you find.

I just did - and wound up with *four thousand, six hundred and forty-three* different items.

Poor Dr. Phil - he's only got four thousand, four hundred and seventy-nine! And Dr. Drew's at a paltry three thousand, one hundred and eighty-six!

Okay, I kid about Doctors Phil and Oz. Obviously, *anybody* would be lucky to have over a thousand related items come up on Amazon. For a doctor to have that kind of marketing firepower is totally awesome.

Of course, until you get your own successful national TV show, those kind of numbers are going to be a

---

little out of reach. What you have to understand, however, is the *concept* behind those numbers.

Doctors Phil, Oz, and Drew are viewed as experts and authorities in their fields - *because they are doctors*. That's why their public trusts in them enough to invest in their books, their videos, their supplements, their diet programs - whatever products they slap their names on.

What I'm asking you to understand is that while you may not have millions watching your every move, *you, too, are trusted in the exact same way by your patients*.

The education and training of doctors, especially in America, is so extensive and rigorous that all of us have a vast array of knowledge at our fingertips that not many others in our society have. And when we don't know something, it's easy for us to find the facts with all the resources at our disposal.

That's a value that goes beyond money. It's the reason patients pay to come to see you - and it's also the reason they'll pay for *your informational products*.

When you give them the information they're after (the 411) - and frame that information in an urgent manner (the 911) - you create products that serve your patients, enhance your value, and grow both your practice and influence.

It's what makes a thriving practice excel.

The Celebrity Product Line

Books. CDs. DVDs. Downloadable audio and video products. These are informational products you can create affordably and easily for your patients. All you have to do is match *their* needs with *your* expertise.

For example, you might regularly treat patients that you diagnose with diabetes - and those patients may have difficulty adapting to the demands of that particular condition. They might, for instance, have difficulty figuring out what they should eat and when. How much they should eat and drink. What kind of exercise regimen they should have in place. In many cases, they probably didn't take good care of their health to begin with, which is how they ended up with diabetes; now, however their life depends on following through with large and difficult lifestyle changes.

That's where you can create an informational product that can help. You can produce a week-by-week - or even day-by-day - guide to following a healthy lifestyle for those afflicted with diabetes. Because you're already their doctor, they'll be comfortable (and reassured) having that kind of assistance from you, even when you're not around.

Of course, there are all kinds of health-related informational products, especially in the diet and exercise arenas, but most of them are fad-related or gimmicky in some way. And the overwhelming majority of them aren't going to be as reliable or extensive as the kind of information a doctor can deliver to a patient.

And, again, there are a variety of ways you can deliver this kind of valuable information outside of an appointment. Your patients can walk away with a simple free brochure that's not really going to give them the detail they may require. But how much better is it to walk out with a prepackaged course on a CD that they can listen to on the car ride home? Or a DVD they can watch in the comfort of their own home?

With today's technology, it's a snap to create these. Your computer is probably already equipped with a video webcam and a microphone. All you must do is hit the record button and talk! Of course, you'll want to do some preparation in terms of structuring the course and bullet-pointing the necessary content so you make sure you cover everything, but it's the perfect way to make a house call without ever leaving your own home!

For Members Only

Another way to build a new stream of income as well as provide additional help to patients is to create a *membership website*. For a monthly fee, patients (and anyone else for that matter) will be given a user name and a special code so they can access exclusive content that you post.

That content can, again, can take the form of video and audio instruction that they can either view on the site or even download. You can also post articles and blogs you either write yourself or are authored by other experts you respect. Another "bonus" is offering to personally answer members' questions on the website, depending on your time availability.

This is an excellent way to build a large "fan base" for your brand. If you consistently provide compelling and useful advice, your membership list will expand beyond your practice - you'll not only attract new patients in your area this way, but you'll also attract members from beyond your practice location.

How? Well, internet users will discover you through Google and other search engines; you might even want to do some online marketing to attract more members once you've posted enough content to make the site look as packed as possible. Social media is another great way to promote your membership website.

As your website picks up members, you'll begin to build a powerful database of names and emails that you can market to in the future, should you write a book or produce a full-length video on a specific topic that you want to sell outside of the website. You'll continue to expand your brand beyond your office and begin to make a national name for yourself.

Putting Your Product Together

You might be intimidated by the idea of creating your own informational product, especially if it's video. You may think it's not for you - because you don't think of yourself as some slick Hollywood on-air talent who knows how to work the camera.

Well, you shouldn't put yourself in that box anyway. You don't *want* to be the guy selling Sham Wow on infomercials at two in the morning - you want to be *yourself,* the same trusted authority that your patients relate to in your examination room. Don't get me wrong, you want to make sure you put some energy into your presentation and that you're articulate about your subject matter - but, at the same time, you should be as natural and relatable as possible, even if it results in some impromptu fun.

For instance, I know a lawyer who began making YouTube instructional videos. He was using a stand-up desk microphone for the audio. Well, in the middle of a ten-minute video, he made a hand gesture and accidentally knocked the mike off the desk.

Now, instead of stopping the video and starting over, he simply said, "Excuse me," to the camera, bent over out of frame, picked up the mike, and replaced it. He then looked at the camera and said, "Now, as I was saying ..."

This ended up being his most popular video - and his most memorable one. A few years after this happened, people still remembered him for it. And believe me, it didn't hurt his business or credibility one iota - this man has built his practice up to such an extent that he's hired other lawyers, so he doesn't even deal directly with clients very much anymore! What it *did* do is humanize him and bond him to his audience.

Whether you're doing a video, an audio-only recording, or just a written article or blog, you may have no idea of where to begin in terms of subject matter. Well, there's an easy way to get started, and it's a method that will undoubtedly spark more ideas.

Think about the questions you're asked most frequently by your patients. Begin writing them down at the end of a day at the office so you have them top-of-mind. Cut that list down to the main ten - and record in detail the answers to those questions.

It's a process that will continue to give you inspiration for more content. As patients come in and ask things about their condition or how they should address a health issue, keep track of those queries and create your content based on the answers.

The value of this is undeniable. As you probably know, many patients can be reluctant to ask these kinds of questions; they're intimidated by doctors. How great would it be for them to get the answers on their own, from you, *without* having to ask?

The great thing about creating these types of informational products is that it becomes another stream of income that's NOT touched by the insurance industry or government regulation. These are also profits you make without having to be "in the room" - as the cliché goes, you make money while you sleep!

Beyond the monetary benefit, you can also feel satisfaction in providing good, solid information to your patients and others interested in what you're offering. Many of the doctors I know complain that there isn't enough reliable information on the internet - people believe anything that some uninformed jerk writes on Ask.com or numerous other "advice" sties.

If you provide the information, it's going to be right. And that alone is worth the effort!

Why You're Worth It

I understand that some of you reading this might feel uncomfortable selling these kinds of products to your patients. It's not exactly what they taught us in medical school!

Remember, you're providing important information to people *who need it*. This is already a huge industry and many of the current products out there need a huge update/upgrade - or a plain old reality check.

And also remember that you worked hard (and spent a lot!) to obtain your high level of expertise and experience. *That's why you should always educate patients about your worth.* When people question how much you're charging for a product or even just for an office visit, feel free to explain to them about the years and the dollars you invested to become the authority you are today.

Now, you don't have to lecture people when you do that. Just be casual and conversational when you relate the facts behind what it takes to become a doctor. There's no need to jump down their throats about something the ordinary person doesn't really think about.

And, by the way, educate yourself about your own worth so you truly *know* your value as a medical professional. You're probably aware that there are lawyers who make two thousand dollars an hour. There are even coaches and consultants who charge clients upwards of $800,000 a year just to provide guidance and information.

So, don't be afraid to charge a fair price for *your* products and *your* time - because there's another very important reason to do that beyond the fact that you're worth it.

People use price to decide level of quality.

You know that when you walk into a Wal-Mart, you're getting a certain level of product. The price is lower - and the quality is lower. However, when you walk into Saks Fifth Avenue or Neiman Marcus, you're in for a totally different experience. You know you're going to pay a lot more for a much higher level of quality. In the consumer's mind, high price equals high quality, low price equals low quality.

Which one do you want your practice to be associated with?

When you charge higher prices, you attract patients that recognize that you *are* worth it. And, as you increase your income, you're able to spend more time and more resources on those patients - which means *their* satisfaction level will climb.

Of course, when you do charge those kinds of prices, you must deliver an awesome experience, as we discussed in Chapter One. However, you'll be able to afford to deliver that experience. One feeds the other, creating prosperity as well as an incredible level of care for your patients.

Creating and Selling Informational Products: Action Steps

As I've suggested, this is one area where you might feel very much out of your comfort zone at the start. The more you do it, however, the more relaxed you'll be and the easier the process will become. Here are three action steps to get you started.

Action Step #1: Mind Your Marketing!

It's true they don't teach marketing in medical school (at least not the one I went to!), but the fact is your practice is as much a business as the neighborhood hardware store and you must attract "customers".

When you're ready to begin creating and selling informational products, you'll need to market them to people. That means you should begin by creating a database of "leads" at your practice. This list of names and contact info should go beyond your list of past and present patients, because, undoubtedly, your informational products will appeal to more than only the people who come to see you.

First, create a website that encourages people to "opt-in." That means you might want to offer a free download of a short "special report" (for example, "5 Steps to a Healthier You" or some other action oriented content that's related to your specialty); you then require whoever wants that download to enter their name and email address (presumably so you can email them with the link to the download, but mainly so you can add their name to your database).

Your website should be set up to automatically store that contact information, so you'll be able to market your products to them when you create them. There are many products that will do just that for you.

Also, create a referral program that rewards patients that recommend you to their friends. This will also expand your database of potential leads. There are also various online services that will allow you to put a referral program into action almost immediately, complete with your own personalized website.

Action Step #2: Go Pro!

You didn't become a doctor all by yourself. You, of course, had teachers and mentors who showed you the ropes.

As this is an entirely new field for you, consider getting a similar level of training from professionals who can help you get off on the right foot. There are smart and experienced marketing and coaching experts who specialize in helping doctors, dentists and other medical professionals maximize their marketing opportunities in powerful, profitable ways that won't embarrass you or your patients.

You also might be looking for some assistance in creating your actual products. For example, you may want to hire a copywriter to help you write blogs and books. You might want a professional videographer to shoot your videos if you're uncomfortable doing them with your webcam set up. And you may even want to hire a coach to help you with your presentation skills. As I said, you don't have to go to these lengths but if you really feel you want the help, go for it!

Action Step #3: Create a Focus Group

Focus groups are used by corporations and Hollywood studios to "test" their output with consumers. Before they spend millions to market their products, they use the focus groups to find out if there are obvious problems that would cause the average person to reject them.

Get your own focus group together for your first informational products! Every doctor has a few patients that he or she feels closer to than others. Ask a few that you trust and respect to look at your first attempts at informational products and get their honest opinions. Avoid asking professionals in television or writing as it's more important to get "normal" people's take on what you're doing, as that's who will be using these kinds of products.

Informational products raise your prestige, your revenues, and your profile. They expand your circle of influence beyond your practice to the world at large. Maybe you won't end up with over 15,000 entries on Amazon like Dr. Oz - but you will end up as a "celebrity expert" in your field.

Chapter 5: DON'T LOOK FOR FISH IN THE DESERT

Imagine if you would a Beverly Hills plastic surgeon who is simply brilliant at what he does.

This guy can literally take decades off the appearances of the rich and the famous - and transform the least attractive of them into completely stunning individuals. And, of course, he charges rates that are through the roof both because of his exclusive clientele and his reputation.

Now, imagines he tires of the rat race that is Southern California and decides to relocate his practice to Buford, Wyoming. Buford, located about halfway between the cities of Cheyenne and Laramie, i.e. the middle of nowhere, consists of a combination gas station/convenience store, as well as a schoolhouse from 1905, a cabin, a garage, and a three-bedroom home.

So - how do we think Dr. Nip and Tuck is going to fare at his new location?

I would bet pretty horribly.

This is a very extreme example of a very simple principle (which is the title of this chapter) - you don't fish in the desert. Because all you're going to catch there is some sand and maybe a case of heat rash.

And yet, many doctors still try. They don't consider where they locate their practice. They don't consider which people they market their services to. And they don't think about what else they might be able to provide to their current patients.

Again, we doctors are not trained to be business people. It's somehow considered unseemly. Ironically, one of the biggest reasons people go into this profession in the first place is because it's an occupation that guarantees a good income.

Let's stop being ashamed of making money. Let's stop pretending that making less is somehow noble. And let's start admitting that the more money we make, the more time and care we can give our patients (and the more we can give back to those who maybe can't afford our services).

Bottom line? More money doesn't mean you're any less of a doctor.

A rising tide lifts all boats - yours, your patients' and your community's. Your prosperity unlocks a lot of opportunities and possibilities for your practice and your patients. So why wouldn't you maximize your income?

It beats fishing in the desert!

Define Your Goals and Refine Your Location

Let's look at the people who make up your practice, as well as the place where it's located. And let's discuss how to maximize the possibilities in both cases.

One of the first things you need to do in this regard is to define what you believe your ideal client's income should be. This is a subject we'll get into greater detail about in Chapter 7, but for now, just know that you need to look for patients who can afford to pay you what you're worth.

We've talked about creating a WOW experience for every patient that comes in. Well, that experience comes at a cost and you need to have people who can afford to help you create that experience.

It's easier to find them than you might think. You can buy marketing lists that identify people by all sorts of demographic information, including income. These lists will help you identify the best and most prosperous areas in which to market your practice and also give you their addresses so you can send your information.

There are also services that will actually dig into your own patient database; they will help you identify your best "customers," analyze their common attributes, and help you identify other prospects that also have those attributes. Those people are more likely to respond to your marketing and join your existing pool of great patients.

This process goes beyond simple marketing, all the way to where your practice is physically located. If your practice is in a working-class area, for example, or an area that's currently experiencing a lot of home foreclosures, that's not a good location. Instead, try to be in an area where people are willing and able to pay what you're asking.

In the last chapter, I asked you to define your own worth. Keep that in mind as you look for the best possible location and the best possible patients. In the long run, that combination brings you the most prosperity.

Dig for Gold in Your Own Backyard

Okay, so you don't fish in a desert. However, you *should* dig for gold in your own backyard.

Why? Well, once upon a time (yes, I'm starting this out as a fairy tale, but it's actually an all-too-true story), a man named R.U. Darby and his uncle caught "gold fever" back in the California gold rush days of the mid-1800's. They staked a claim in the area close to places where the precious metal was being mined and they quickly went to work with a pick and a shovel to determine if they had lucked into a fortune themselves.

A few weeks and a lot of sweat later, the men finally found some gold in the ground. Joy! Happiness! And another challenge. They needed the massive mining machinery that would bring the ore out of the ground in large amounts and put big money into their pockets. They traveled back east to tell their other relatives the good news and asked for some investment money for that machinery. As they were trusted good men, they got the stake they needed.

With the machinery, they began bringing up the ore and for a short time, everything seemed great. But suddenly, they couldn't find any more gold. They dug and dug and dug with the heavy machinery, but couldn't find the vein of gold that should've been readily available.

Their money and their willpower finally ran out. They sold off the machinery for pennies on the dollar to a junk man and also handed over the claim. Well, the junk man knew about gold and knew the veins of the metal traveled in a straight line. He found the big strike they were after *only three feet* from where the Darbys had decided to call it quits! That meant he made millions while the Darbys went bust. Instead, they spent years repaying the people who had entrusted their money with them.

This is a famous story recounted in Napoleon Hill's groundbreaking book, "*Think and Grow Rich*." Darby, who learned his lesson, lived the rest of his life as salesman who was persistence personified. He would never take "no" for an answer, because he remembered that tragic moment when he did quit - with a fortune sitting only three feet away.

The moral of the story was pretty obvious to Mr. Darby and hopefully it's apparent to you as well. There is a vein of gold to be mined right in your own "backyard" - aka, your practice - and that's from your current patients. You're not going to realize that fortune, however, unless you go about trying to "mine" it in the right way.

The Payoff from Your Existing Patients

Here are a couple of important facts from Forrester Research: it costs 6 to 7 times more money to get a new customer than it does to retain an existing one. The same study also showed that a company can also boost its profits as much as 95% - simply by retaining at least 5% of their current customers.

Switch out "patient" with "customer" and "practice" with "company" in the above paragraph and see if that doesn't rock your world.

Obviously, you must continue to market to new patients, using the guidelines we just discussed; but, even more urgently, you want to hang on to the ones you have, especially your core group of "premium" patients.

"Premium patients?" you might ask. "What's that all about?"

Okay, let me explain. I already made a passing reference to your "best patients" but here's where we're going to get into more detail about who those people are. There's a business truism called "The Pareto Principle" (also known as the "80/20" rule). That principle holds that most businesses realize 80% of their income from 20% of their customers. Translated to medicine, that would mean that roughly 80% of your fees come from 20% of your patients.

Now, this is meant only as a rule of thumb, which means your numbers probably don't break down in a perfect 80/20 split. You will undoubtedly find, however, that a core group of your patients is the bedrock of your practice's prosperity.

If you can identify these patients, the ones who come in the most and always pay without a problem, you've hit a vein of gold. These are people who already believe and trust in you, who will probably gladly refer you to their friends and family and who are the most likely to buy the additional informational products you create that we discussed in the last chapter.

When you give them the proper attention, when you encourage them to refer you and to purchase additional products and services from you, you'll find your income from them rising even higher - IF you market to them correctly.

So, you want to make sure these people know about your informational products, if you are creating them. You want to make sure they know about your membership website, if you've built one of those. You also want to make sure they know about all the services you provide, even if they're for something they hadn't thought to seek treatment for.

As you remind them of all these things, also remind them that these are all provided by you so you can maximize the wellness of each and every patient who comes to see you. After all, it's not as if you're selling t-shirts with your logo on them or anything (at least, I hope you're not!). You're providing real value to improve their quality of life.

You and your staff should always spend some extra time and care with these special "premium" patients. They should feel like honored guests at your offices - because they really are. Just as Frequent Fliers get to wait at the special airline lounge at the terminal, you should pamper your best patients as best as you can.

The Other 80%

But what about the rest? What about that 80% that may not currently be your vein of gold, nonetheless, are still patients who pay for your services?

Don't ignore them. Because you never know.

When I go shopping here in America, I am often not treated like someone who has substantial buying power. I'm an African-American woman and, depending on the store I walk into, a salesperson might never even approach me to see what I'm interested in.

If I feel I am deliberately being dismissed like that, I walk right back out.

Why should I patronize people who don't respect me enough to find out what I'm all about? It's a foolish assumption. I'm attractive and well-dressed; might it not be possible that I've got some power in my purse?

I had a completely different experience in Hong Kong when I walked into a high-priced watch store. They knew I was an American and assumed I did have money, so they were all very nice to me - not over-the-top nice, but very respectful and helpful. I picked out a watch, I went to pay for it and I pulled out my Platinum American Express card.

That's when things changed in a hurry.

There was a mirrored wall to my left - and apparently, it was a one-way mirror. I was being observed and my exclusive card was spotted. That wall unexpectedly opened-up and the store's management came out to see what else I might be interested in. When they saw the Platinum card, they realized they had undersold me and of course, were anxious to rectify that little mistake!

The point is you don't know the buying power of each and every one of your patients. You may have some that come in for the occasional check-up and you don't really think about them that much, but they could be in need of some other products and services that they could pay for easily and willingly.

So, yes, pay extra attention to your best patients. But, if you are doing anything extra with your practice, take the time to make sure ALL your patients know about it. You don't know who might be interested in it and who can afford it!

The fact is you don't know where the buying power is. American singer, Sean Combs (P Diddy) created and marketed his own premium brand of vodka because he knows the African-American community has a lot of buying power, even if the majority of American businesses dismiss that power. If you write off a person because of his or her race, you may be writing off a great patient.

And if you think appearance or wardrobe is the ultimate arbiter of how big a bank account, just remember that Howard Hughes, one of the richest men in the world at the time, walked around in jeans and dirty tennis shoes.

Oh yeah, and he didn't trim his fingernails either.

Your staff should be trained to help pay attention to all these patients; again, your time is limited. But, when you do have appointments with them, take a little extra time with everyone to find out more about them.

Pumping Up Your Practice Power

When you leverage your location and the quality of your patients as much as you can, you leverage your own value to that of a thriving practice. Here are three important Action Steps to get you started:

Action Step #1: Diagnose Your Demographics!

As we discussed, location is critical to becoming a thriving practice. Unfortunately, when most of us were starting our practices, we didn't really think about where we were putting them in a business sense. We just wanted to get our medical careers going as best we could.

Well, it's never too late to reevaluate your location. Just as an expensive restaurant can't make a go of in a rundown area, an upscale practice isn't going to fly where free clinics get most of the business. Think about your goals for your practice and whether your location matches up with those goals.

There are professional marketing companies that can help you look at what the demographics of your area are and, if the results aren't to your liking, they can also help you find a good alternative. Ideally, you want to move somewhere close enough for your existing patients to still be comfortable coming to appointments, but far enough away to appeal to a new and more prosperous area.

Like much of life, it can be a balancing act, but one well worth the attempt.

Action Step #2: Pamper Your Premium Patients!

Keeping in mind the 80/20 rule, you want to make sure your core group of best patients "feel the love." That means you may occasionally want to send them a voucher for a meal at a good restaurant or a gift card to an upscale store or something that thanks them for their business in a meaningful way. You can also try to give them little bonus gestures of consideration, such as scheduling their appointments in a way that minimizes their waiting time.

What you don't want to do is call attention to this special care so that other patients recognize and resent it. Obviously, you want to be working to give all your patients a great experience but some will deserve a higher level of consideration.

Action Step #3: Information, Please!

Some of the 80% who aren't your "premium patients" could join that elite group if you find out what makes them tick. You and your staff should identify the occasional patients in your database and make a note that, the next time they come in, you or they will conduct a more thorough Q and A with them to determine more of their overall health needs and goals.

When you're armed with that information, you have a much greater chance of success marketing products and services that are matched to their specific needs. You also increase your level of engagement with them and vice-versa.

Many patients don't think twice about leaving a practice simply because they believe the doctor really doesn't care if they come and go. The more you show your interest in them, the more you bond them and the more value you can provide to their lives.

And that's something of a legacy.

Chapter 6: HOW TO HAVE AN INAPPROPRIATE PATIENT RELATIONSHIP

Okay, don't be afraid of this chapter because of the title, I'm not trying to get you sued for sexual harassment or anything.

What I am trying to do is teach you how to keep *patients for life*.

There's a reason that I still remember the name of Dr. Ann Madigan, even though it's been a whole lot of years since I've seen this woman's face. She was my son's pediatric dentist and she was very important when my boy Xavier was three, because he ended up knocking out a tooth and needed a temporary replacement in there until his adult tooth came in.

But that's not why I still remember her name seventeen years later.

I remember her name because every year, after I took Xavier to her, she would send him a card for his birthday. Years after we moved out of her practice area, she kept sending him a birthday card. You can bet that if I ever had to refer anyone to a pediatric dentist in that area, the name "Dr. Ann Madigan" would immediately fly out of my mouth just because she made this very small gesture that cost her very little in time, effort and expense to remind me of who she was.

In the first chapter, we talked about how to make your patients love you. Well, passion is fleeting (which is why the divorce rate is so high!), so in this chapter, we're going to focus more on how to keep your relationship with your patients fresh and alive. Some of the suggestions I offer here may strike you as "inappropriate" for a doctor-patient relationship, but, believe me, they are essential for a Doctor who wants to build the strongest and most prosperous practice.

Keep 'Em Coming Back for More

Before I forget, we're going to talk about reminders. Bad joke, intentional.

Reminders are an obvious way to get patients back into your office for another visit, no matter what your specialty is. Everyone needs a follow-up at some point and every doctor needs to make sure their staff sets up another appointment with a patient down the line before they're out the door.

Then, of course, before that next appointment, you remind them about it. Stunningly obvious. What's not so obvious is what the best way to deliver that reminder is.

For instance, email seems fast and easy, right? Best of all - completely free! Everybody uses it, so why not?

Well, in my case, I'm looking at my inbox and there are currently 30,000+ messages sitting in it. Now, I will admit I'm not the best at cleaning out that inbox, but the fact is people get so many emails these days that yours might easily get lost in the overload.

Also, consider the fact that many overzealous spam filters could throw your email directly in the trash and email becomes even more problematic.

I'm not saying don't use email, but use it as more of a back-up for your reminders. Your marketing always needs to stand out from the crowd and that can be hard to do in an overcrowded inbox that's filled with marketing messages from stores and other vendors.

The fact is that everything old is new again so remember the good old U.S. Post Office. People's email inboxes may be filled with junk, but their physical mailboxes are very lonely places and an opportunity for your reminder postcard to make the desired impact.

There's also another advantage to using the regular mail for reminder cards and other communications; it helps you keep current on where your patients are. When you use "Address Service Requested" on your mailings, you'll be able to keep your system updated on changes of address. You'll also get back mail that can't be delivered, meaning you can either mark patients down as "inactive" or try to hunt them down wherever they may be so you can attempt to reactivate them. You want your staff to keep your patient database as clean as possible, so you don't waste money and effort mailing things out to addresses that are no longer valid.

Finally, consider using the latest technology to really make a reminder hit home. There are call services that will physically phone your patients with pre-recorded reminders and also ask them to confirm appointments by hitting numbers on their phones' keypads, requiring them to make a response in the easiest possible way.

Texting is another powerful way of sending a reminder because it's direct and one-on-one. When you receive a text on your mobile phone, you instantly check it out because what if it's from someone important? Well, your text just put YOU at that same urgency level so you can almost guarantee that your reminder will be seen. Again, there are automated systems out there that can make text reminders a breeze for you and your staff.

Special Events - Special Results

Let's face it, sending out reminders is all about business. Most patients are cynical about them - "Oh, they just want me in there again so they can get more money out of me. They don't really care about me."

That's exactly the attitude you don't want in your patients. That's exactly the attitude that makes it easy for them to dump you for another medical provider at the drop of a hat when it's convenient for them.

That's why special events can bring you special results.

You have no reason to remember or recognize special events in their lives. Whether you're a dentist, a chiropractor or a cardiologist, why should you care? There's nothing in the doctor-patient relationship that requires you to send out a birthday card.

Oh, but patients looooove to get those cards!

Remembering Dr. Ann Madigan's example, I sent out birthday cards to my patients. My staff didn't get it at first. "You're spending a lot of money on this. And it's a pain in the neck. Why?"

Because it made patients understand that I really cared about them. And it wasn't that expensive. If you send out postcards instead of conventional greeting cards, it's very affordable.

Especially when you calculate the value of a patient for life. That's what things like birthday cards help you get. If a birthday card to a patient helps you keep that patient coming to you year after year - well, that more than pays for all the birthday cards over the years, and then some!

But if you really want to show a patient how much you care, don't stop at birthdays. Make note of other significant events in your patients' lives.

Just make notes on their charts when they discuss an upcoming major wedding anniversary, for example, or a child's high school graduation, and send them a card on the big day. If you happen to find out that someone special in their lives has passed away, be sure and send something. In this instance, you don't want to just send a card, but a gift basket or something more substantial, such as a contribution to the charity of the deceased's choice, if one has been specified.

At the very least, under these kinds of difficult circumstances, express sympathy for the person. I have a friend who had been seeing the same gynecologist for about twenty years. She had been married about the same amount of time. Well, sadly, her husband had recently died from cancer when my friend went in to see the gyno for a scheduled appointment. She told the doctor that her husband was dead. The gyno merely replied, "Oh yeah, I heard something about that," and then said nothing more about it. Not even an "I'm sorry."

Well, that was the end of that twenty-year-old relationship. She dropped that doctor because he seemed cold and callous about a devastating incident in her life.

You must care about the people you treat in order to be the best in your field. It's an investment that simply must be made.

The Name Game

An important part of the respect you show a patient is simply finding out how they like to be addressed.

Doesn't it annoy you when you say to someone, "Call me such-and-such" and they call you so-and-so instead? What's the point of asking if you're not going to listen?

So, when you do ask, make a note of the answer as soon as you can. Make it a part of their records and make sure the staff knows as well. Always err on the side of being formal. Use the last name and "Mr." or "Ms." in front of that last name.

You want to make sure people are as comfortable as possible with their ongoing relationship with you. If you can't even be bothered to call them by the name they prefer - well, how's that going to work out?

Answer? It's probably not!

You can even offend someone, depending on their culture and values, by addressing them incorrectly. For example, when an African-American woman is older, you don't just use her first name. When you call a seventy-year old "Annie" instead of "Miss Annie," it's considered very disrespectful.

If you think I'm making too much of this, let me tell you a story about a medical colleague that I liked. I referred a patient to him and she was an older African-American woman. He simply called her by her first name all during the appointment.

He was an excellent doctor and gave her top-of-the-line care, but all I heard from the woman's daughter was the fact that "He called my mother by her first name!!!" Everyone has different value systems that's why you ask the question of what they want to be called, and that's why you keep a "cheat sheet" with the answer in their file.

Here's another great system that can help you and your staff put names and faces together; when a patient comes in, take a quick picture of them and stick it in their file. Have your staff review the pictures of the patients coming in that day so they can greet them by name when they walk through the door.

And be honest about it when you ask to take their pictures. Have your staff tell patients that they want to make sure they know who everyone is, because it is a big practice and many people only come in every year or so.

All of this may seem like overkill, but again, I'm a doctor who has plenty of horror stories about other doctors lousing up this simple show of respect. Here's another one. My dad needed eye surgery, so I sent him to a doctor I knew and respected. Once again, I believed this guy would take care of my father and give him the personal attention I expected.

Well, after the appointment, the doctor called me up to tell me what he thought should be done. And his diagnosis was fine. What ticked me off, however, was the fact that he kept referring to my father as a "her." It was "She needs this kind of procedure" and "Her sight could be affected by this."

My dad suddenly became a transgender case.

And it's not like my dad has a name you could mistake for a woman's like Tracy, or Lynn or Terry. No, his name is Kenneth.

I sent a note to his office saying this was unacceptable and he called me to apologize. But this completely blew my mind; how could you make that kind of mistake? Especially when you're talking to the guy's daughter, who's also an eye surgeon??? Again, the care was top-notch, but what lingers was the fact that the doctor couldn't keep my dad's sex straight.

In Chapter 1, we discussed how patients sue doctors mostly because there's a bad relationship. An actual medical mistake may be accepted, if the doctor actually shows concern to the patient and the family. I have another doctor friend who got sued, but they had trouble seating a jury because she had such a great reputation in her community. The case finally ended up with a hung jury and a mistrial largely because they liked her so much.

In contrast, the opposite is also possible. Maybe the doctor didn't make a mistake, but the family ends up hating him or her to such an extent that they sue anyway!

You don't have to be Oprah and you don't have to be Hitler either! Show your best face to your patients and wait until you get home to yell about the tough ones.

Your life will be easier and your practice will be better for it.

Secrets to Long-Lasting Relationships

The stronger (and longer) your patient relationships are, the more "fans" you'll have out there in the world singing your praises. Here are three great Action Steps to help you achieve this.

Action Step #1: Soup Up Your Staff!

We can't do it alone! That's why you must make sure your staff is trained to interact in a positive way with everyone who walks into your waiting room. Your support staff is the face of your practice and in many cases, your patients are interacting with them more than they actually interact with you.

With that in mind, make sure that when you hire people, they have pleasant personalities and your interaction is good during the interview. Also, invest in some training for them in catering to the patient relationship and doing what has to be done to keep patients happy.

You want to make sure your staff is so good the patient would miss one of them if they weren't there. Hell, they should be so good, you should miss them too!

And when you do accidentally hire a bad apple (it happens all the time), look at whether it's possible to retrain or re-educate them, or if you need to get rid of them. If it's the latter, retain an expert in employee law and make sure you're following the right process for termination.

Action Step #2: Cheat with Abandon!

Earlier in this chapter, we mentioned making a "cheat sheet" so you'd know how to address a certain patient. Well, the cheating doesn't have to stop with their names! Consider creating cheat sheets with not only their names, but also such relevant personal information as the names of their children (and ages), their spouse's name, whether they have any pets, what they do for a living, if they have any interests - basically, any stuff about their life that they feel is important enough to talk about. That way, you and your staff can quickly review that before their next appointment and show your consideration by asking questions like, "How's it going with your new car?" or "Did your daughter get that scholarship?"

You won't believe how your patients' faces will light up when you do.

Action Step #3: Reward Referrals!

If you don't have a referral program in place, you're missing out on a big opportunity and wasting all the investments you've made in building up your patient relationships. When you've gone to all the trouble of creating a WOW experience for people and you and your staff have made an effort to create long-lasting bonds. You create a group of advocates for your practice, as we discussed in our chapter on branding.

Take advantage of that enthusiasm for you and your services and put in place a formalized referral program, just like your cable or satellite TV company would offer. Reward patients who refer a certain number of new patients your way with a suitable gift card or restaurant voucher and let them know you appreciate their recommendation.

When you create an inappropriate relationship with your patients in the good way, mind you - you create something infinitely stronger than the usual doctor patient interaction.

And that's something you can take to the bank!

Chapter 7: PATIENT ZERO (AND YOU'RE LUCKY IF IT'S ONLY ZERO)

We've been talking a lot in this book about all the things that go into creating a thriving practice; providing informational products, developing amazing experiences, being seen as the expert in your field, and so on.

But now let's get down to it. I'm talking dollars and cents. The bottom line.

You need to know how much money you're making on every single patient and plan accordingly in order to build your practice to where you want it. Many doctors are just breaking even. They've got a whole practice filled with Patient Zeroes. Some doctors even have a bunch of Patient Minuses, with days that actually cost them money rather than earning it.

When it comes to your ROI, you want everyone who walks into your offices to be a Patient Plus.

This chapter is all about working the numbers in your favor, so you can serve your patients at the highest level possible. It's also about the delicate matter of making sure you collect your fees from those patients in the most effective but diplomatic way possible.

Most people try to avoid talking about money but you've got to if you really want to be the best of breed. Let's talk about the ways you can make your practice profitable and give the best care to your patients.

The Cost of Being the Boss

Before you can talk about your numbers, you need to know what those numbers *are*. That means identifying all the costs involved in operating your practice on an average day.

The first step is adding up all your annual expenses - INCLUDING YOUR SALARY. Pay yourself first because you're working hard and you're obviously the backbone of your own practice. Now, include the cost of your offices in total - staff, the space itself, taxes, and so forth. Everything you can think of. Yeah, I know it's scary - but do it anyway!

Now, divide that figure by the number of days you're in the office per year (in other words, vacation days, holidays and weekends don't count because you're not making money then). That number is your average daily cost.

The next step is to figure out how you're going to meet that cost or, hopefully, exceed it.

That involves how many patients you need to see throughout the year, based on the different procedures you offer and the fees you charge for those procedures. You need to include the average number of revisits per patient after a procedure and so forth. Obviously, all this will be determined by your specialty and the services you offer, so you, or ideally your staff, must determine the parameters here.

The number you're after in this process is *the average revenue per patient*. When you balance that with the number of patients you see per day, you'll get an idea of whether you're making more than your average daily expenses, making just enough to cover them, or, horror of horrors, making *less*.

When you have all those calculations, you can finally answer the all-important question: Is the person walking through the door a Patient Zero, a Patient Minus or your ultimate goal, a Patient Plus?

Making It All Add Up

If you need to ramp up the revenue, happily, there are a lot of ways to make that happen.

First, look at what gives you a higher profit margin. In many cases, it may not have anything to do with what medical service you provide. You may not know this, but most movie theatres don't make their real money on ticket sales, they make it on the ridiculously overpriced snacks and drinks they sell.

Similarly, when I was an eye doctor, my profit on selling glasses was MUCH higher than what I was paid for performing cataract surgery on a patient. Not only that, when the patient was looking at frames and trying them on, they weren't taking up any of my time.

My staff handled those kinds of sales completely on their own.

There are other things along those lines that you can sell. People today are very interested in maintenance and preventive services. What can you sell in that arena that dovetails with your practice? It could be as simple as skin products or supplements that you legitimately believe in.

Also, think about either trying to do more of a certain kind of high-end procedure or offering an entirely new procedure that's more profitable than what you're currently providing. For example, a lot of dentists these days are performing Botox injections, along with their more traditional Novocain ones.

When someone wants to improve their looks, they're willing to pay a heftier price for the results they're after and dentists may be more aware of that fact than any other medical professional, except for plastic surgeons, of course!

Beyond Botox, dentists already understand the power of selling cosmetic dentistry procedures and products, which is why you'll see those things heavily marketed, not only to young people, but also to older patients who may have been recently widowed or divorced, or who need to look better to find a job or get a promotion.

These types of products are highly attractive and highly profitable. When you can expand your offerings in this area, you expand your profit potential so don't be shy about selling them if you have them. For instance, use "Before" and "After" pictures to demonstrate how dramatic the difference can be, so patients understand what the benefits are.

Your Staff Is Your Sales Department!

At many practices, doctors will pay for their staff to get sales training, especially those employees who answer phones and interact most often with patients at the office.

The reason? They often have to act as salespeople, whether they understand that fact or not.

For instance, when a person needs a medical professional in your area, and they call your practice to ask questions about you, your staff person needs to know how to engage that person in a conversation and not just answer questions with a "Yes" or "No." They also need to at least perform the *minimal* marketing task associated with that kind of call ...

getting the person's contact information!

We discussed in earlier chapters the importance of building a marketing database. This is the perfect opportunity to add to it. A person who calls your practice is what's called a "hot lead" - *someone who's already interested in your services*. Why on earth would you want to throw that info away?

Here's another good question: why would you ever waste a chance to sell *other* products and services to the people coming in and out of your practice every day? Your assistant should be trained to be on the lookout for patients with other problems to which you can offer solutions.

This isn't some sleazy marketing scam, by the way. As I'm sure you're aware, sometimes, those patients *simply don't know to ask* - because they don't know everything you can do for them. But a patient in need is a patient you should heed because when you can provide them with relief to a problem, they'll be glad to take it.

And here's another big secret.

Don't sell procedures, sell benefits.

That's why we talked about "Before" and "After" pictures earlier, what better way to show the benefit of something?

Of course, sometimes the benefit of a medical service is avoiding a lot more trouble down the line. Your patients should always be made aware of the consequences of doing nothing. Hit the pain points so they understand what could happen if they opt out of taking action.

Don't get bogged down in detailing a procedure, service or product, unless there are specific points they need to know. You and your staff should always focus on outcomes, so that patients understand what "the big gain" will be from investing in what you think they need.

Collect Your Fee - Without Losing the Patient!

You know how to get really stuck with a Patient Zero? When one *doesn't ever pay you!*

Whatever way you bill your procedure, you always need to collect what you're owed.

I encourage doctors not to take insurance, I also encourage those who do to collect the co-pays up front, before the actual appointment begins. There's a huge reason to do this. If you're slack on collecting those co-pays, the insurance company can actually decrease your fees by the amount of the co-pays that you're owed if they decide to audit you. They will end up discounting your fee - and, long-term, that is a pretty brutal blow to any practice.

Now, let's talk about the office person that you designate as the one who's responsible to collect all those fees. That person has to have certain people skills or bad things can quickly happen with good patients.

For instance, a friend of mine was in the middle of switching insurance companies when she went in for an appointment with her doctor of several years. She was unaware that the coverage of one policy had lapsed before the new one began and the office had simply collected the co-pay as usual. The appointment went as planned and she went home.

A week or so later, she got a nasty call from the doctor's office. "Did you know your insurance didn't cover your last visit?" She was surprised and said no, but she wanted to check into it to make sure before she paid the $200 that wasn't covered. The person snapped, "I'll send you the bill," and hung up.

A couple of weeks later, the woman went back in for a follow-up. She had received the bill, but had not paid it yet. She usually took care of those things at the end of the month. The person who had called greeted her at the desk. Maybe "greeted" is the wrong word, she *assaulted* her. "You're not getting in to see the doctor until you pay this bill in full."

My friend was incredibly insulted by her manner and very embarrassed that she was being yelled at about a two-week old bill in front of other patients in the waiting room. She said, "I don't know if I'll ever want to see this doctor again," and she turned around and walked out.

She never went back there again.

None of that drama would have happened if the office person had treated her nicely from the start. As it happened, the approach was all about anger and distrust from the start, and for no apparent reason; my friend was a patient in good standing and had always paid whatever she owed. Why immediately treat her as though she was some kind of deadbeat?

Asking for money is always a sensitive situation. Of course, getting payment upfront is the best way to prevent any kind of disagreement (and if you do take insurance, maybe you should have your staff check to see if the patient's policy is valid on the day of the appointment!). But if people owe you, there's a right way and a wrong way to handle it.

It starts with asking, "Can you take care of this today?" NOT DEMANDING.

And, if it is a patient you like, and they are having financial troubles, as so many are, ask if they can at least pay a portion of what they owe. Be nice and respectful. As I mentioned in Chapter 5, you never know what a patient's real buying power is.

Billing Do's and Don'ts

Again, I do strongly advise collecting payment upfront. Make that payment as easy as possible for your patients by accepting all the major credit cards (even American Express, even though their fees are a little higher).

If you get payment upfront, you also avoid the expense of sending out bills. It can cost you four to ten dollars to send out a single bill and that shouldn't be necessary. Whether someone goes out to buy groceries, or a car, payment happens before the product changes hands. Your services should be no different.

There are a couple things you can do, however, when you DO have to send out a bill. Use bright pink or blue paper in an envelope that has a window. Believe it or not, the color catches people's eyes and it causes them to pay the bill more frequently than a bill that's printed on white paper. File that under things you didn't know!

When you are put in a situation where someone has owed you money for a long time, you may have to hire a third-party collections agency. I understand the problem, but for me, personally, I think it's an ethical problem to use aggressive collections tactics on patients.

What we used to do is use a company that would send out a series of letters, starting off pleasantly, and then getting progressively firmer, using language like, "We appreciate if you have a dispute with the bill; if so please contact the doctor's office to resolve it. Otherwise, please pay the balance by such-and-such a date or we will have to report this outstanding balance to a credit agency."

This was an effective tactic for my practice; we never threatened to go after anybody's firstborn child, we just stuck to the facts and let them know where it was going to go if they didn't pay.

Yes, you want your money, but you must look at the lifetime value of the patient in question, especially if they're going through a short-term financial problem. Be fair, but tough.

And again - *collect upfront!!!!*

Here are a few Action Steps to turn your Patient Zeroes into Patient Heroes.

Action Step #1: Fire Problem Patients!

Yeah, I know, I know. I just talked about why you should be extra-nice to patients and extra-understanding when they can't pay.

But, I have to be real here. Sometimes, life gives you bad patients. They keep coming to you, even though they act like they hate your guts. They make your staff miserable. They don't pay on time even when they can afford it. And they're a lot more trouble than they're worth.

Well, life is too short for anybody to be unhappy and that includes both them and you. You could spend that time on another patient who is glad to have you as their doctor and wants to work with you. The problem patient is what I call a "drainer." They drain your resources, your spirit, your time, and your finances.

You must be very diplomatic when you fire them. You might just tell them that you have another colleague who might treat them more effectively. You should even take the time to introduce them and try to make the transition as smooth as possible.

Action Step #2: Improve Payment Strategies!

If you offer a lot of high-ticket services, always use an *outside* finance company to allow your patients to make the big purchases even if they might not have the funds on hand. The advantage of using an outside company is you get your money and collecting is that company's problem. You avoid conflicts with your patients.

There are also other ways to help your patients pay their medical bills. For instance, San Diego-based Sharp Healthcare improved payment by giving their patients tools to navigate federal and state payment support systems at registration.

I'm not sure what economic conditions will be like at the time you read this book. What I can be sure of is that the more you help out patients with payment options, the happier both you and they will be!

Action Step #3: Script Your Staff!

As I said, whether they know it or not, your staff also function as salespeople - especially when they take incoming phone calls from people interested in coming to the practice.

Professional marketing agencies often supply actual phone scripts for medical staff, to help them properly engage with the person calling and to present your practice and its services effectively and in the most attractive way. When your staff follows a script, all talking points are covered and, most importantly, the caller's contact information is gathered.

Script your staff for success or, at the very least, get them the basic sales training they need to do their job correctly.

Every day, you should be checking to see how much revenue you made that day from your patients and how that stacks up against your average daily expenses. Every day, you should be checking to be sure you're making the income you need to support your practice properly.

This isn't just about boosting your bank account. When you increase your revenue per patient, you gain a better lifestyle and your patients get a better level of care. You won't have to overbook appointments to make enough money, and you won't have to feel rushed or stressed, running from exam room to exam room to take care of everyone throughout the day.

Instead, your Patient Zeroes will turn into Patient Pluses and, better yet, they'll realize big pluses from your practice. You'll be able to spend more time with them and create deeper relationships with them.

Better care. Bigger revenues. What more could you want?

Chapter 8: A PATIENT IN NEED IS A PATIENT YOU HEED

"You never know until you ask."

It's a familiar saying, but its wisdom is all too often *overlooked*. Think about the many life situations where we court failure by *not* asking about things we need to know. When we don't ask, when we continue on blissfully unaware, not fully armed with the facts, reality, at some point, crashes down on us, leaving us to wonder, "What happened?"

Relationships, business deals, major purchases - when we neglect to find out the information we need, we end up making bad *decisions*.

Your practice is no different. We need to amend the saying slightly to ...

"You never know what your <u>patients</u> want until you ask."

If you want to serve your patients better AND your revenues to increase (the two goals that should go hand-in-hand for every medical practitioner), you need to properly identify your patients' needs and be responsive to them.

And the only way to do that is to, yes, ASK!

Survey Says ...

More and more companies are becoming increasingly aggressive about getting customer feedback on their service. I'm sure that you have had the experience of contacting a business about an issue, and then immediately getting either an email or a phone call from their customer service department, surveying you on how well the business performed in responding to your need. The best restaurants and hotels *always* ask for your opinion after a visit.

The big boys of business don't do *anything* full-out like that unless there's something in it for them. Customer satisfaction surveys not only tell companies what they might be doing wrong; they also, if constructed correctly, tell these same companies how *they can make more money.*

Think about how many times you've seen a survey question that begins with the words, "*Would you be interested in ...?*" As in, would you be interested in these kinds of products, these kinds of services?

As in, *would you buy more from us if it was something you needed?*

Surveys may seem like a trivial tool for your practice, but they can help it in two important ways. First, they can help you pinpoint problems or holes in the WOW experience you're trying to create for your patients. Second, they can identify crucial patient needs that you may not be meeting.

When you construct your survey, you want to make sure to have those two parts in place. When your patients are leaving your offices (the best time to hit them, when the visit is still fresh in their minds), you want to ask for:

1) Their Testimonials

Your survey should ask questions like, "What did you think of the care you received at your appointment?" "How could the experience have been improved?" "Was the staff courteous and helpful?", as well as anything else that is relevant to your specialty or practice.

By the way, this information is not only useful to the ongoing improvement of your practice, it's also helpful to your marketing efforts. If a patient gives you an amazing testimonial, you want to be able to use it on your website or in other marketing materials.

Make sure to have a box on the survey form that they can check that gives you permission to use their kind words wherever you want. Odds are, if they're that effusive about you and your staff, they won't flinch at giving you that permission (remember Brand Advocacy from Chapter 2!).

2) Their Needs

In this section, you want to ask them to identify other areas of their health that they're concerned about, where they might need additional help and/or resources from your practice, and what they feel is currently lacking. Also, ask if they would like more information on a particular condition they have or more guidance on something *outside* of your practice.

Make these questions as open-ended as possible, to prompt more thoughtful answers.

What you want to look for in those answers are trends or a consensus forming around something that maybe you *should* be offering, but aren't at the moment. That could be anything from commercial products related to your specialty (for example, as an eye doctor, I got suggestions from patients to offer a particular brand of eyeglass frames) to a new procedure or extra medical service (for example, a dentist who doesn't offer orthodontics might have patients who'd like that service, so it's more of a "one-stop shop" for all their dental needs).

We've spent a couple pages on the benefits of a survey but that doesn't mean your survey has to have the thickness of the old Yellow Pages book. You need only five to ten relevant questions that address the above two areas. You don't want the survey to be a long and arduous affair. It has to look like a quick and easy task to the patient or you're bound to hear complaints.

You may hear one or two complaints anyway. You may have to eliminate a couple nonessential questions, but continue to ask your patients to fill out the survey in the post-appointment period. It's important to learn as much as you can about how your patients relate to your practice. You'll also find that patients are much more willing to reveal opinions in writing that they might not be comfortable saying to you in person.

Not knowing these opinions, again, can be harmful to your practice's health. When you get the same answers from several patients, that indicates something you need to pay attention to, whether it's good or bad.

Don't Leave Your Patient "Home Alone!"

One of the things you may find out from your survey work is how you can continue to help patients *outside* your offices. For example, in Chapter 4, we discussed how newly-diagnosed diabetic patients might appreciate an informational product that could help them adjust to dealing with their condition. We also talked about created a "members-only" website that might contain enhanced content that your patients (and others) could have access to for a monthly fee.

Again, you can deliver this information through audio, video, or written blogs and articles over the internet. You can also sell CDs that are accompanied by a transcript of the information on the discs, or DVDs that feature you, on camera, explaining a condition.

These tools allow you to make "house calls" without actually going anywhere, and deliver expert and reliable information that your patients might otherwise have trouble obtaining.

As you are probably aware, websites are teeming with medical misinformation that could cause much more harm than good. By providing an alternative that your patients can trust, you're extending your reach beyond the examination room and into their daily lives, meeting their ongoing health needs in a major and impactful way.

These information products don't have to be filled with hours and hours of material. The best way to approach this is to offer relevant advice, in short and easy-to-digest chunks that don't overwhelm the patient.

It's easy to create these audio and video products yourself, using your desktop or laptop's microphone and webcam. However, there are other tasks that are often a part of this process that you will likely want to "outsource" to others who have the time and the talent to get them done.

This is where the internet once again comes in handy. There are several websites that will help you give these products a professional polish that will burnish your brand and impress your patients. Here are a few online resources you should be aware of:

- **Fiverr.com**

Fiverr.com is a site where you can really make some amazing deals that's because everyone is offering to do stuff for literally *five dollars*. You might find someone who can do a cover design for a book, DVD or CD, for example. There are a lot of people on this site offering to do a lot of different things (many of them completely crazy, but they're entertaining to read!) and they just might spark some thinking on your part on how to give your informational product an extra burst of creativity!

- **99Designs.com**

If you're looking to create a new logo or business card, revamp your website design or create any sort of graphic for an informational product, 99Designs is another valuable resource. Here, you can get a professional end product at an awesome price - because the artists and the designers on the site "audition" to do your job, and you pick the person with the best ideas for your project. The site has set prices for design work, usually several hundred dollars.

- **CreateSpace.com**

CreateSpace.com allows you to create professional-looking CDs, DVDs, and books which they then manufacture strictly to meet demand. That means you won't have cartons of books out in your garage waiting for buyers. This is a great done-for-you service, especially if you want to sell your products on Amazon and other online retailers. CreateSpace.com has all the resources you need to help you design and put together a professional completed product.

- **Upwork.com**

When you want a lot of written content provided for your website, Upwork.com has a vetted group of quality writers to provide it at a discounted cost. They can deliver large, complex projects that ordinarily might be too expensive when done through traditional means.

- **Upwork.com**

Upwork.com also plays host to the world's largest group of online freelancers who provide an incredible range of services. Whether you're looking for a writer to help you generate written content, a web designer and/or programmer to help you create your dream website, or a graphic artist to provide the perfect look for a product, this is the best place to look.

Simply post the description of the job you want done and your price range, and freelancers will immediately start "bidding" for the job. Be aware that many writers are based in such countries as India and Taiwan, and may not provide the best level of English. By the way, the biggest companies in America have fallen prey to this, as illustrated by this actual email a friend of mine received from AT&T after he complained about something:

"Thank you for taking out time to contact AT&T. I sincerely apologize for the inconvenience that you have experienced. I will defiantly assist you with all your concern and get back to enjoying your day further!!"

Yes, that was a cut and paste from the email! In most cases, you can avoid the above almost-English by reviewing the freelancer's past feedback and portfolio. This will allow you to make a good assessment of their abilities and their suitability for your job.

The Art of Autoresponders

Autoresponders are another valuable way to stay in touch with your patients between office visits. If you don't know what autoresponders are, they're simply prewritten emails that are programmed to be sent out to a recipient on an automated basis. They can be strictly educational or they can sell a product or service in addition to the education. The education content is the key, though, because you're providing *value* to your patient (and at no charge).

For example, in an autoresponder, you might talk about a procedure that patients may be unaware of that can treat a condition or solve an ongoing health problem. At the end of the autoresponder, you can mention that your practice offers this procedure and to contact your office for more information. You can even do a series of autoresponders educating the patient about the procedure, outlining more of the benefits in detail.

You can also use autoresponders to reach out to potential *new* patients, if you've built up a good database of names and emails for marketing purposes (as I discussed at the end of Chapter 4). If you offer free downloadable content in exchange for a person's email address, you'll find yourself rapidly building up that database and, with the power of autoresponders, you can immediately start marketing to anyone who leaves their contact information.

To give you a better idea of what autoresponders are like, here's a typical one used by a dental practice that's hoping to increase their implant patients:

SUBJECT HEADING: *Your Free Information*

Hi {FIRST NAME},

Here's the link to your free Special Report on "7 Important Benefits of Dental Implants". Click on the link to start your download:

www.YourDownloadLinkHere.com

I also wanted to share with you, a story from one of my patient's that's very relevant to the information you'll be receiving. I don't know what your current situation is, or if you have an ongoing problem with dentures or missing teeth, but, recently, one of my patients shared with me how getting dental implants affected his life.

****

Wade (that's not his real name, it's been changed to protect his privacy) said he always dreaded losing his teeth as he grew older.

The reason? His mother lost her teeth at an early age. Eventually, she had no options except to use dentures. Wade could see, however, that the dentures didn't really replace the comfort, stability, and usability of her real teeth. She couldn't chew like she used to and her face began to age more rapidly, due to the loss of bone tissue.

Wade didn't want the same thing happening to him. So, when he ended up losing two teeth to cavities, he asked us what the best option was to replace them. We told him dental implants were a great permanent solution. They maintain the bone tissue, give you up to 90% of the chewing power of real teeth and don't require a lot of extra care. And no messy adhesives.

Wade had the implants put in. And he told me that they worked so great that he would never consider any other treatment for missing teeth.
By the way, his mom is still with us and she's getting implants to support her dentures next week.
****

That's one of many similar success stories we've had at my practice. If you want to find out if implants are right for you or someone else you know, we are offering a limited number of free consultations. Just call us at (PHONE NO.) and we can make an

appointment to simply discuss what options are
available to you, without pressure or obligation.
It only takes a phone call to change your life!
Committed to your dental health,
{DENTIST NAME} {PRACTICE NAME}

As you can see, the best tone to strike with autoresponders is a friendly and conversational one. You don't want to send out a hard sell email with your name on it - that won't go over well!

You also don't want to stop at one. Sending out a *series* of autoresponders is important because, as most professional marketers will tell you, prospects don't usually buy on the first contact or even the second. You want to know how many times it usually takes? It takes *17 contacts* to make the sale! This isn't to say you need to send out 17 autoresponders to the same person but it does mean that follow-up contact is vitally important to your efforts.

Create Powerful Bonds with Your Patients

If there's an ongoing message that you should be learning from this book, it's that the more you do for your patients, the more they'll do for you. When you find additional ways to serve them that go beyond the doors of your practice, you'll become a regular presence in their lives and they'll feel bonded to you in a more meaningful way.

Here are three Action Steps to help you do just that:

Action Step #1: Look at What You're NOT Doing!

Start compiling a list of products and services you're currently *not* offering that others in your area of practice do offer to their patients. To create the list, confer with colleagues, ask in online forums where other medical professionals participate, and check out the websites of practices similar to yours to see what they offer.

Cut down the list to products and services you would be comfortable selling to your patients. Make the list a part of your patient survey and ask those taking the survey to simply check off which ones they might be interested in. This will give you a good indication of which are worth adding to your "medical menu."

Action Step #2: Total Up Your "Touches!"

A "touch" refers to every occasion where a patient or prospect encounters your name, either through seeing an advertisement, noticing a post by you on social media, or through direct contact via a phone call or email. As I mentioned, marketers say it takes up to 17 of these touches to clinch a sale with most people.

Review the many ways you are currently reaching your patients outside their normal appointments with you. Are you using social media regularly? Autoresponders? Does your staff follow up with patients who haven't been in to see you for a while?

Make sure you truly are a presence in your patients' lives and that they have every opportunity to "reach out and touch" you. Have your staff "friend" your patient list on Facebook, for example, to make sure you're connected with everyone you should be connected with. Finally, see if you can hit the magic "17" number with all your various touches.

Action Step #3: Video Your Patients!

Consider keeping a video camera handy at your practice. Why? Because video testimonials have a great deal more power to them than written ones and it's very hard to deny the plausibility of a real person saying real things on camera.

If someone you've treated has responded remarkably to your care in ways that have improved their life dramatically, ask them if they'd mind talking about it on camera. Again, you don't need a professional video crew to shoot these things, just point the camera at the patient in your office and ask them to talk about how your treatment helped them. You can even make it into an interview, especially if they're a little shy about talking.

Think about giving the patients that agree to a video a little gift as a "thank you." You want them to feel appreciated and not exploited.

When you work hard to meet your patients' needs, you'll find they end up taking care of your practice's needs. Find out what they want and deliver what they want. That's the modus operandi of your thriving practice!

Chapter 9: YOU'RE A DOCTOR - DEAL WITH IT!

I was shopping with my husband for our upcoming wedding (we had already been legally married and now, we were about to fly to Rome for a big church wedding) at a quality department store. My man needed a tie and I instantly saw the perfect one. I said to him, "This is a fabulous statement."

He looked at the price tag and made a few statements of his own.

The fact was, I had zeroed in on the most expensive tie in the place, $260 worth of tie. And even though there was a giant sale going on in the store, the tie was not included in the discounted goods.

I turned to the sales guy, put on my best smile and said, "Everything else around here is on sale and it's Father's Day (which it was). Can't you give us a break?" The sales guy frowned and said, "I really can't, I could lose my job if I did."

"Just a little break?" we tried again.

Well, as we walked over to the cash register, the wonderful sales guy slapped a sale sticker on the tie and took the price down to $155.

Now, most people won't even try to negotiate in a store like this. They see a price and they pay that price and they don't think they really have a chance to get it down. But the fact remains, *the store wants to make that sale.*

And there's always room for negotiation!

Why Doctors Need to Deal

If you look at extraordinarily successful people, one of the top traits they have in common is that they're *great negotiators.*

Donald Trump, who wrote the world-famous best-seller, "The Art of the Deal," is the prime example of this. He started doing big real estate deals before anybody else was doing them and he did them in difficult times. His team always had a mandate to make the deal happen on Trump's terms. Some of his deals even required changing zoning laws and those laws got changed to accommodate his wishes. Why? *Because the cities in question wanted the deal to happen.*

Just like our department store wanted to sell that tie. The bottom line is that the other party always has needs they want to fulfill in the deal, too. You are usually not the only one who wants a deal to happen and, in most cases, the person or company you're negotiating with has that very same desire.

The only way you're ever going to find out if you can make the deal you want is to ask, ask, *ask!* And when you do ask, ask for the moon and the stars. If you only get the sun, you'll walk away happy!

Now, how does this apply to medical professionals? Why is knowing how to deal such a big deal for your practice?

Because *you should negotiate with patients and businesses every day.* You may not like it and you may not want to admit it, but it is a critical aspect of your practice.

The harsh truth is that doctors usually don't even like to *ask* in a negotiation, because we think it's somehow beneath us. We don't ask for things from insurance companies, from our patients, or from our office landlords. And, let's be real, if you don't even ask, then it's not really a negotiation, and it's the other guy who ends up getting what he wants instead of you.

Let's talk about how you can be a doctor who deals.

Negotiating Your Patient's Health

There's a two-step process to successful negotiating. The first step is to sit down and *think about what you really want* out of this negotiation. Have that focused clearly in your mind and again, don't be afraid to ask for everything you want. You always want to go in high, to give you room to cut down your wish list when push comes to shove.

The second step? Try, whenever possible, to make your idea seem like it's the other guy's idea. When the person you're dealing with comes up with a potential solution on his or her own, that indicates they've already invested themselves in the situation. By carefully crafting your approach, you can make at least some of what you want seem like something they want.

Let's talk about how you can accomplish this with a difficult patient. Maybe this person isn't following a diet and exercise regimen and or taking the proper medication for a condition when necessary. Whatever the case may be, if you truly want to help, you must *successfully negotiate*.

See how important this skill can be?

You have to give your patients choices. Let them know the benefits and costs, in terms of their health. "If you do this, you get better. If you don't do this, this bad thing happens."

As you talk to them, you want to spin it and lead them into giving you the right answer, so they make the best choice for their health. Now, let me be clear, I am not talking about being dishonest with a patient or lying to them in any way. You always want to operate with integrity in a patient consultation.

However, it is *still* a negotiation to get patients to do *what is in their best interests.*

Let me give an example. There are certain conditions which are better helped by non-pharmaceutical means and one of them is depression. Now patients may want the quick fix of a pill, but many studies show that patients with depression end up doing better simply by making positive changes in their lifestyles rather than taking the latest anti-depressant. When they get out of their shells and interact more with other people, it's a big help, in most cases.

But, again, patients today just want to feel better *now* *H*ow do you help them to a long-term solution that will be healthier for them?

Maybe you talk about the side effects of medication. Maybe you also talk about another patient with depression who took yoga classes and began to feel better. And maybe you've *negotiated* a deal with a local yoga studio - they give you first-class-free coupons and you feed them a steady stream of new clients. Maybe you mention that that other patient started yoga because of the coupons you have. And maybe this patient says, "Well, I guess I could try it. It would be better than being on those pills forever ..."

And suddenly, it's *their* idea. They're more invested in following through.

Now, this isn't going to work every time, but, for the times it does, that patient is going to come back with a new appreciation of you. They got better without pills and the dangerous side effects and because you offered a viable alternative.

The Prescription for Getting What You Want

Let's move on from patients to business negotiations. Dealing with an insurance company or a contract on your office space can be stressful situations, no doubt, but they're both still negotiations, which means you must begin by asking for what you want. Because most people don't.

When I was considering moving on from my practice, I wasn't sure if I was going to keep my office open but my lease was about to expire. I called up the landlord and said, "Look, we need to keep the terms the same for the next year." He said, "Well, I don't know if I can do that." I said, "Well, I'm going to move out if you don't."

I won that negotiation!

You must be tenacious and you have to let the other party know you're serious. If you are having problems getting an insurance company to agree to something, then ask for their supervisor. If they still won't budge, ask for *their* supervisor. And just keep going. You might not get exactly what you want (i.e. the moon and the stars), but they might come up with a good alternative on their own (i.e. the sun), maybe even one that's better than what you asked for in the first place.

When you don't let up, they'll usually step up with some kind of solution. Which is better than nothing.

Tapping into Trump-Style Negotiation

I've laid out some important broad strokes for your negotiating tactics, but I would also suggest you check out the book, "*Trump-Style Negotiation*," for a more in-depth look at this subject. The book was written by George Ross, who has put together Trump's biggest deals over the past thirty years and helped him make billions of dollars. Ross provides a lot of great insight that has certainly helped me develop my skills.

Here are a few more tips from this master dealmaker to keep in mind during your next negotiation, along with some more comments from me:

- **"Build trust, friendship, and satisfaction with the other side"**

Being nasty usually isn't going to get you far. The other party won't want to deal with you on a human level and may even actively look for ways to screw you without you knowing it (think of the diner who yells at the waiter, who then spits on the guy's food before he brings it out to the table). Instead, work at building trust and a genuine concern for the other person.

This, of course, is especially important to do with your patients. When they trust and feel comfortable with you, they're more likely to take your advice.

- **"Discover what the other side wants, determine their weaknesses, and uncover valuable information"**

Remember what I wrote when I was talking about getting the discount on my husband's tie? *The store wanted the sale.* They didn't want us to walk out without buying that tie. The weakness, in this situation, was that practically everything else in the store was on sale. And in my lease negotiation? When I let the landlord know I was more than willing to walk out the door, he quickly folded. Always use whatever you have and whatever you know about the other person to your advantage.

- **"Convince the other side they're getting more than they expected"**

The best way to conclude a deal is with both sides believing they've won something, even when, in my landlord's case, all he won was me staying another year at the same price!

- **"Use timing, deadlines, deadlocks, and delays to your advantage"**

Let's go back to our patient with depression that we want to treat without medication. If we really want to encourage that patient to do something like the yoga classes, we could say, "Well, I'd like to wait until your next visit to prescribe something. In the meantime, ..." and then, make some suggestions on lifestyle changes they could put into action. By delaying the prescription, you create the space for them to try something new.

When you can control the pace or progress of negotiations, you create maneuvering room for yourself that can really pay off in the end.

- **"Become an expert on the topic you're negotiating"**

If you're going to negotiate with an insurance company, learn their protocols and procedures to the extent that you can forcefully and reasonably argue your case. When you just demand things without knowing if they can be provided, the other side gets frustrated. When you speak knowledgably about their side of the negotiation and their challenges, they feel as though you're taking their situation into consideration (while, of course, you still go after what you want!).

- **"Be flexible and consider multiple solutions to every impasse"**

As I wrote earlier, during a negotiation, when one of your requests seems impossible, the other side may come up with an alternate solution that could work just as well. Don't dismiss these suggestions out of hand; consider them and even propose some of your own. Be creative about what you want to do. Flexibility is crucial to a successful negotiation; if you don't give, you don't get.

The Real Meaning of No

There's one last important point I'd like to make about negotiating - and that's when you end up hearing the dreaded word, "No" from the person you're dealing with.

First, a "No" isn't forever. *It just means "No" at that moment.*

If you have small children (or even big ones!), you know what "not taking 'no' for an answer" *really* means. You tell a kid he can't have any more candy or you can't take him to Disneyland or whatever else he wants more than anything on earth. And they don't stop. *They will keep coming back until they wear you down.* They'll whine, they'll yell, they'll ask in different ways, they'll butter you up, they'll give you options …

Yes, in short, kids are master negotiators. Watch a four-year old go to town trying to close his deal, and you will soon realize that fact.

If your kid keeps asking for something until he gets it, *shouldn't you?*

Let's say, again, you're negotiating with an insurance company. They say, "No." Okay, so wait. The optimal time to be able to go back to someone and ask again, without being perceived as being a pest, is about ten days. If you wait that long and ask again then, it's going to seem more like you're keeping in touch, rather than nagging.

You can be persistent without being a pain. You don't want to be a four-year old, but you do want to win. Keep going after what you want. You'll be surprised how often you get it.

Sharpen Your Negotiating Skills

Want to be the biggest deal-making doctor in your town? Here are three action steps to get you on your way to negotiating success:

Action Step #1: Identify Wants vs. Needs!

When you're negotiating, make a list of "Wants" and "Needs." The difference is important. Obviously, you *have* to meet your needs and that's the whole reason for the negotiation. Your wants are a different story, however; those are the things that it would be nice to have, but aren't essential to closing a deal.

Never sacrifice needs for wants. For example, you wouldn't walk away from the car of your dreams just because they didn't throw in tinting the windows.

The other crucial aspect to this step is to also make a list of what you think the other side's wants and needs are; understanding those gives you more power. For example, my landlord *wanted* to raise my rent, but he *needed* me to stay to keep the cash coming in. I assumed that is why I won the showdown.

Action Step #2: Hear What They're Saying!

Listening is an art and it just might be the most important negotiating skill of all. If you dominate all discussions and never give the other party a chance to explain themselves, you (a) make them angry and (b) miss out on learning some important information that could help you. With many people, the more you let them talk, the more they say that they maybe shouldn't. Let them talk and talk for as long as they'll go. You might be surprised at what you end up finding out.

Action Step #3: Practice, Practice, Practice!

It's time to start your negotiating residency, doctors! That means working on your negotiating skills outside your practice. Here are a few tasks you should attempt:

- Try to negotiate down a fixed price at a store, as I did with my husband's tie.
- Successfully talk a friend or family member out of something they want and get them agree to something you want and try to make it seem like it was *their* idea.
- Call your cable or satellite TV company and say the cost is too high and you're going to

disconnect it. See if you can renegotiate your monthly rate.

- Identify a patient who's going out of his or her way to *not* do what they're supposed to do for their health. Make it your mission to talk them into doing it.

Deal-making is a crucial skill for all parts of your life; that means working on the techniques and tactics in this chapter will help you get more of what you want more of the time. Remember, a thriving practice wouldn't be caught dead losing out in a negotiation!

Chapter 10: TIGER WOODS NEEDS THEM - AND SO DO YOU!

Now, you may be thinking there are a few different ways to read the title of this chapter, in terms of what Tiger Woods needs, given his scandal-laden past. Rest assured, we are keeping this clean.

Despite his ups and downs in recent years, Tiger is still regarded as one of the great golfers of all time. Given that track record and his many years of accomplishment, you would think the man knows everything there is to know about the game.

Well, he doesn't think so. Because Tiger Woods still has a coach. Oh, wait, that's wrong. He has *three* coaches, because this is a man who is intent on staying on top of his game for as long as possible.

Those who achieve the most don't stop trying to grow in their abilities and their knowledge, and they know they can't stay in their own personal bubble to make that happen. They constantly search for input from the outside, from other successful people, to continue to learn new tricks and techniques that will take them even farther in life.

And they always make sure their foundation stays strong.

Legendary UCLA basketball coach, John Wooden, who coached that team for almost 30 years and won 10 NCAA titles in 12 consecutive years, always had an interesting first step for his players at his first talk of the season. It probably wasn't so interesting for the seniors to hear the same first talk they heard when they were freshman, but Wooden was a man who believed in the proper process, which is one big reason he was voted "Coach of the Century" by ESPN.

That talk was all about Wooden demonstrating, in meticulous detail, how the players should properly put on their socks and their shoes. Yes, he *would show them how to do it.*

Why? Because Wooden knew that too many good players ended up on the bench because of blisters that formed during game play. He knew most of those blisters could be prevented *if players would simply take the time to correctly put on their socks and shoes.*

A great coach will take you back to those baby steps to move you to a place that's more advanced than you ever thought possible. That's why having a coach is the secret for all doctors who want to achieve awesome things for their patients and for their practice.

Who's Masterminding the Store?

We'll get into individual coaching a little later in this chapter, but first, let's talk about the power of Masterminding.

Most of you reading this book know about the power of Grand Rounds sessions for medical professionals. When multiple doctors get together to discuss difficult patient cases, everyone benefits from the shared knowledge of many medical minds (especially the patients!).

A Mastermind group is no different when it comes to building a powerful practice in every aspect. When you associate with other successful doctors, you make *yourself* more successful.

Your medical Mastermind group should center on the *business* of your practices, something the rest of the world doesn't really like doctors to talk about but, as we've emphasized in this book, when you succeed at the business end of your practice, you are able to provide a higher level of care for your patients, as well as give more back to the community.

But, because the public doesn't like the words "business" and "doctor" to ever intersect, all the people in your Mastermind group should sign a confidentiality agreement stating that nothing discussed inside the room will leave the room. There's also another, even more powerful reason for all of you to keep quiet. The insurance industry could actually accuse you of anti-trust action!

In general, Masterminds can work exactly like a Grand Rounds. Each doctor can put themselves in the "hot seat" to hash out an ongoing problem at their practice. The rest of the doctors can then weigh in on the issue and offer their solutions.

Think about starting your own medical Mastermind group. You can do it in one of two ways; you can either make a point of only inviting doctors who have specialties that don't conflict with yours, or you can include competitors in your Mastermind group, if you have a perspective of abundance (i.e. there are enough patients to go around for everyone).

Which would I suggest? Well, when the practices represented in a group are the most similar, then the solutions that are suggested will be the most effective. Your number one priority is to do the best by your patients and that should be your goal. It may be most productive to stop looking at practices like yours as competitors and begin looking at them as partners.

Of course, your Mastermind options also depend on the size of the community you're serving. By the way, if you do practice in a smaller town where there aren't many other doctors nearby, consider using teleconferencing or Skype conference calls to carry out Mastermind meetings with doctors in other areas.

The Power of Individual Coaching

Masterminding is a cooperative effort. That means everyone wants to get along, even as they help each other optimize their practices.

Coaching is not so cooperative. It's more about finding the right person to *kick your butt.*

This isn't to say you're not good at getting things done. Obviously, you became a doctor and that's certainly far from the easiest thing in the world to achieve. However, when you want to build your practice with a Billion Dollar mindset, it requires an effort and a focus that goes beyond your day-to-day doctoring, not to mention your private life.

The truth is, to truly find ultimate success, you must rededicate yourself in a way that's going to be difficult short-term, but amazing in the long run.

It's kind of like when you know you should lose weight. You know what you have to do, but sometimes, it isn't a lot of fun. So, you eat those three donuts in the kitchen. You blow off stopping at the gym on the way home. And then, when you step on the scale, you find out just how badly you've let yourself down.

Who really gets punished when you stop trying? You do.

That's why, when you want to build your practice with a thriving mindset, you need someone to make sure you follow through and turn *thought into action*.

The right coach will understand how to help you build a successful practice, keep you on track and, most importantly, *hold you accountable for achieving your goals*. If no one is looking over your shoulder to see if you're living up to what you need to do, it's all too easy to let things slip by, over and over again, until you find you're going backward instead of forward.

You wouldn't be reading this book if you wanted that scenario to play out.

When you were on your way to becoming a doctor, you always had coaches and mentors that you could learn from and ask for advice. They were your teachers, your professors, and the doctors you encountered in your internships and residencies. For some reason, though, most doctors stop looking for that kind of leadership when it comes to their own practices.

Thus, those practices don't live up to their potential.

You put a coach on your payroll to avoid that dead end. That coach isn't there to be nice. He/she is there to hold you accountable and push you forward. What you must always remember is that the coach is there to promote *your* best interests. To help you reach *your* goals. To get you to where you said *you* wanted to go. The coach isn't making up your future for you. He or she is trying to help you fulfill the one *you* desire.

Let's face it, there are very few bad doctors because our standard for becoming one is so high. However, almost every doctor is a bad *businessperson,* simply because they're not expected to concern themselves with dollars and cents.

That's why doctors need to have a coach or mentor who *KNOWS BUSINESS.* Trust me, I practice what I preach. Recently, I was negotiating a contract and my coach was an invaluable help to that process. He gave me an objective viewpoint of what I needed to attain and how to reach that result. He saw things I couldn't see, because I was in the middle of the situation. As an outsider looking in, he had no emotional involvement that might impair his judgment.

Let's go back to Tiger Woods. Or even you, if you golf. If you're hooking your swing to the right, a coach can see what you're doing and tell you how to correct the problem. On your own, you wouldn't know what to do to fix your swing, because if you *did* know, you wouldn't keep on hooking to the right!

Your coach will have solutions to problems that you haven't thought about. These are solutions you can't get from a book or a webinar or a seminar, because those solutions are not specific to your issues.

In contrast, your coach knows exactly where you are and what you want to accomplish. He or she is so close to you that you can be transparent about everything that's happening in your life. You can be honest about everything with your coach and that coach, in turn, can give you honest and *actionable* feedback.

Three Coaches for Success

I really believe people should have three types of coaches or mentors in their lives; **a life coach, a business coach, and a spiritual coach.**

These are very different disciplines and require very different types of expertise. That's why you want to make sure to get very high-level people to coach you - people you *know* are true authorities in their area.

For example, the pastor at your church might be the obvious choice to be your spiritual advisor, but he or she might not be the right choice. The pastor may be young and relatively inexperienced and not understand your personal challenges.

You also will want someone who is well-trained in the coaching arena. For instance, you might think a psychologist or psychiatrist would be the same thing as a life coach, but they really aren't (and apologies if you are one of those!). A therapist will try to lead you to your right answers; it's more of a listen-and-comment process.

That's not what a coach does. A coach will actively give you recommendations for achieving your goals and won't be afraid to tell you what's right and what's *wrong* about the way you're going about reaching those objectives.

A life coach helps you achieve balance in all things. You'll want to discuss all areas of your life with him or her. Those include your finances, your relationships with your spouse, your parents, your kids, and your friends, your leisure time activities, your health, and your involvement in your community.

If any *one* of these areas is affecting you in a powerfully negative or time-consuming way, it's going to throw things off-balance - and it's going to affect how well you perform as a clinician and a business owner. If you are not performing fully, then you are doing a disservice to your patients. That's why it's probably more important that a physician have a life coach than many other occupations - and yet, so few employ one.

A business coach, obviously, will bring you focus and clarity when it comes to your business activities. I'm not just talking about your practice here. I'm also talking about other business ventures, such as investments. The more financially sound you are, again, the better you will perform your medical duties.

A spiritual coach is not just someone you might pray with, it's someone who helps you sort out your own beliefs and how they fit into your life and your work. Maybe you're an atheist, so you're saying to yourself, "Well, why in the world would I need a spiritual advisor when I don't believe in God?"

Well, think about this situation - what if a patient turns to you and asks you to pray for them?

There are always issues and scenarios that a doctor encounters that fall into the spiritual realm. You want to have the highest possible ethics when you deal with these cases and the right spiritual coach gives you the guidance to do that.

"Put Me In, Coach!" - Three Action Steps to Up Your Game

Pro athletes are far from the only people that employ coaches. So do the world's top CEOs. As the world grows more complex, coaches give us the objective insight to navigate the increasing number of minefields we walk across on a daily basis, so that we arrive safe and sound at our desired destination.

Here are three Action Steps you should take to ensure you get coached to success:

Action Step #1: Make Masterminding Your First Coaching Stop!

When you make the decision to embrace coaching, the best place to begin is a Mastermind group. It's a great way to begin to see what setting goals and being held accountable to them is like; a successful Mastermind group will inspire you to want to move into individual coaching.

Most top-level professionals combine Masterminding with individual coaching; that way they have multiple people to call on for different life situations. Most of them have found the cost is well worth it, because their incomes have grown by leaps and bounds because of those coaching resources.

Masterminds aren't free. The cost is about $10,000 to $25,000 on the low end, which will usually include three or four weekend sessions a year, where the group physically gets together. There is generally a Mastermind leader who takes questions by email to keep things going in between those meetings.

Top business people happily join these groups, because they want to be able to connect with people like them. In their day-to-day lives, that doesn't happen very often. In business, they're usually dealing with competitors or subordinates, and can't comfortably compare notes with people at their level or even above their level. And because everyone is paying that kind of money, all participants will take the group *seriously.* Plus, you get exclusive access to some brilliant secret strategies that just don't get made public.

Action Step #2: Vet Your Coaches Before You Hire Them!

You can't call yourself a doctor unless you have the right credentials. You won't believe (or maybe you will) how many people call themselves a coach even though they have no real qualifications for doing so. That's why some people consider coaches a joke. When someone who can't make a living any other way suddenly declares that they should be in charge of your life, you tend to want to laugh in their face.

You need to ask a potential coach if they've graduated from any kind of recognized coaching course. Who do they coach? Will they supply references? Do they have a strict code of ethics, one that you can actually read? What type of programs do they have in place? And beware - if they aren't clear about the financial end of their services, they may show up with a surprise bill with several more zeroes on it than you expected.

Be wary of the charlatans and search for the real thought leaders. It's easy to tell the difference if you take the time to look closely enough.

Action Step #3: Make Sure Your Coach Majors in Chemistry!

Individual coaching is an incredibly personal process. When you're one-on-one with a coach, sharing the most intimate and confidential information about your life, that coach must be someone you feel confident with and trust. Otherwise, you'll hold back and your coach won't have all the necessary information to properly guide you. That, in turn, will frustrate your coach and accelerate a negative cycle that does neither of you any good.

That's why you must make sure your coach majors in chemistry, that is to say, chemistry with *you.* You should be able to tell whether you have a connection with a coach in an initial meeting or talk, by throwing out a few opinions about your life and your work and seeing how they respond.

If this sounds like a "first date," you're right. You're exploring the potential for a real relationship with this person - and you want to be sure that's possible before things "get serious." If you don't click during your first meeting, that's a bad sign for what's to come, so sit down with some other possible coaches and keep searching for the right choice.

Let me conclude this chapter by saying three big words - YOU NEED HELP. I mean that in the nicest way possible, because I'm no different. There were periods when I went through rocky times in my practice, when I didn't know if I could pay my bills, times when a coach would have helped me immensely.

Nobody does it all on their own. The people that are the best and the strongest in their fields are the people that don't stop learning, growing, and pushing forward. We doctors spent a lot of money going to college and medical school and we barely survived the economic strain of our internships.

So - you're not going to continue to invest in yourself?

That's unfair to your patients - and it's unfair to you. Thriving practices love to be coached because it's the secret to success!

Conclusion

This book was designed to help you (and any other medical professional) consider a "reboot" of your practice from a business perspective.

I even call it a Billion Dollar perspective. Why? Well, as I've mentioned elsewhere in these pages, billionaires think very differently – and their success is a direct result of their mindset. It's not the way we doctors are taught to think.

But it's time we did.

When billionaires position themselves, they create powerful brands that leverage *visibility* and *credibility* in multiple channels; channels that, in turn, can create passive and recurring income streams.

In other words, time is no longer linked to money. They don't have to continually *work* to *earn*. They enjoy better lives and better *lifestyles* by branding themselves in this way.

For example, Donald Trump probably makes more money from licensing agreements than he does from real estate deals. He licenses his name to luxury hotels and resorts, and gets well paid for books, TV shows and personal appearances - all because he has a brand that makes money without him having to actually do much of anything.

Similarly, Martha Stewart has her name on her own magazine as well as everything from Christmas ornaments to cleaning solutions – products that she has very little to do with. However, her brand allows her to expand into these areas that are compatible with both her image and her expertise.

Moving closer to the medical field, you can look at the examples we've used in this book, people like Dr. Phil and Dr. Oz, who have a great deal of credibility and visibility from their media work, and therefore, can command big fees just for showing up somewhere.

Now, you, the person reading this book, may have more impressive credentials and higher degrees than Dr. Phil and Dr. Oz. But their resumes didn't build their brands – their marketing, their systems, and their media savvy did.

What doctors need to understand today – and what is NOT taught in Medical School – is that a doctor who is better at marketing, who creates an awesome patient experience in his or her offices, and who establishes the necessary levels of credibility and visibility will have *more* success that all the other doctors who may have higher clinical skills and/or better credentials.

That understanding is complete when doctors also understand that, if they're going to remain successful, *they have to stop being the cook.*

When you stop being the cook, you stop being trapped in the kitchen and making all the meals for customers. Instead, you stand back and create a string of five-star restaurants that generate income as well as bolster your brand.

You become Gordon Ramsey. Hopefully, without his temperament – I don't think anyone wants to be a patient at "Hell's Practice!"

Think of brands like Saks Fifth Avenue and Apple. These are companies that have an incredible brand – and incredible customer systems in place. Even Wal-Mart leapt ahead of the competition because of the way it marketed itself, not because what it offered was somehow superior to K-Mart or any other discount department store.

Here's the bottom line: Today's medical marketplace demands that you need to work on your overall business strategy, not just your clinical strategy. To do that successfully, you must be able to answer the following questions about your practice:

- How is your practice different from everyone else's?
- Are you marketing yourself as the unique authority in your specialty, as well as the ideal and only solution to your patients' problems?
- Are you creating a "world class experience" at your practice? Do you have the "Wow Factor"

in place that will create a loyal "tribe" of patients – patients who will happily pay your fees, become your advocates, and refer their friends and family members to be part of your "tribe?"

- Are you thinking about how to create alternate and complementary streams of income that will provide extra value to your patients (and allow you to invest more into serving them at a higher level)?

The answers to these questions will assist you in building a powerful brand that will help you deliver better service to your patients as well as create the foundation for you to develop ongoing success in the face of continuing health care economic issues.

This may be the end of this book, but it should be the start of the thought process that will ultimately transform your brand and your systems to a more successful model.

Towards that end, I invite you to visit my website at www.RichDoctorCoachingwww.HelpMyPracticeSucks.com for a free Special Report I've created for that purpose. It's called "The 10 Steps to Start Building Your Billion Dollar Practice Today," and you can download it at no cost whenever you wish. It's my "thank you" to you for having purchased and read this book.

In the meantime, I wish you all the best with your practice and hope that one day you, too, will be able to proclaim, "MY PRACTICE ROCKS."

Congratulations!

It is time to first celebrate your victory. You created a goal of finishing this book, and now you have accomplished it. It is very important to take time, even if it can only be a moment, to celebrate your victories.

Recognize that you are one step closer to reaching your vision. Know that we are proud of your success and very grateful that you took the time to learn and consider how you are going to implement our teachings.

Your next step is to nurture these lessons and then take massive action!

"Inaction breeds doubt and fear. Action breeds confidence and courage. If you want to conquer fear, do not sit home and think about it. Go out and get busy."

~ Dale Carnegie

www.ingramcontent.com/pod-product-compliance
Lightning Source LLC
Chambersburg PA
CBHW051213170526
45166CB00005B/1875